# SONPOLLO

# DRUGS SEX & PROTEIN SHAKES

In Pursuit of the Perfect Body

## JOSEPH SHIELD

**A Sonpollo Book**
**Published by Sonpollo Publishing**

NEW YORK    LONDON    SYDNEY    SINGAPORE

## SONPOLLO

Copyright © 2014 by Joseph Shield

First Sonpollo Edition 2015
For information about special discounts for bulk purchases, please contact Sonpollo Special Sales:

info@josephshield.com
www.josephshield.com

Manufactured in the United States of America

*"An eloquent and well-researched deconstruction of the male body and the perils of self-objectification: as lean and sinewy and oxygenated as the muscles that inspired it"*

**- Ian Kerner NY Times best-selling author of 'She Comes First'**

# WARNING

The following content contains explicit material and explores themes that may cause offence. The themes explored in 'DRUGS, SEX & PROTEIN SHAKES: The Pursuit of the Perfect Body' include: body image, sex, sexuality, drugs, love and violence.

The content presented within this book is likely to challenge your existing views on life, and may cause you to question and reflect upon your own thoughts and behaviours.

# ACKNOWLEDGMENTS

Thank you to all of my friends and family who have offered their invaluable support and guidance throughout the writing of this book.

In particular I would like to thank Professor Lisette Burrows, from Otago University, for her continued encouragement and support. Your enthusiasm, knowledge and expert advice has helped make this journey possible.

Finally, I want to acknowledge all of the young men who participated in my research. Your openness and honesty of your experiences, has provided a rich source of information that has helped to shed light into your unique lives and the various influences that have contributed to your sense of self, which many young men and women will be able to relate to.

Thank you to you all.

# CONTENTS

# CONTENTS

# PREFACE

In a world obsessed with beauty, self-image, 'selfies', celebrities, and looking good, a well-groomed, athletic and sexually desirable body has become a valuable asset. Everywhere we look there are advertisements showcasing beautiful, desirable and sexualized images of young models, sports stars and actors enticing you to buy the latest product. These often- provocative images quickly attract our attention; make us stare, and gaze, as we become seduced by their seemingly flawless aesthetically pleasing physiques.

Many of us wish that we embodied such a perfect body ourselves - the thick hair, the perfect smile, pristine white teeth, silky smooth skin, an athletic physique, and jaw-dropping abdominals. However, it's not only their bodies that we are envious of. We want everything that they seem to have, everything that is associated with having a beautiful body – more sex, the perfect relationship, the dream job, fame and fortune. We only need to look at Kim Kardashian or any other young Hollywood actor or actress to see what physical perfection can get you.

The connection between the perfect body and the perfect life, portrayed though advertisements and the mass media, has influenced our subconscious minds and shaped the way that we experience our own bodies and think of and treat others. Research suggests that the more attractive you are the more you will be liked and admired. Consequently, many of us - subconsciously and consciously - will do whatever it takes to create a desirable body of our own. Whether you like it or not we have been socially conditioned to monitor, check, and scan our bodies constantly for any physical imperfections, blemishes, and flaws to make sure that we live up to our own, and society's, expectations.

For those who feel that their physical appearance doesn't measure up to the social ideals that surround them they are likely to become highly self-conscious about the way they look and experience feelings of anxiety and physical inadequacy. In an attempt to fit in and to feel better about themselves many will look for quick fix solutions so that they can 'treat', 'cure' or cover up their perceived imperfect body. For many of us this process has become a daily ritual. For many of us, creating and maintaining a desirable body - the quest for physical perfection, is perceived to be an essential process that we must undertake if we are to achieve our dreams and get ahead in life.

Whilst looking good clearly has its advantages, such as attracting the attention of others, flirting your way to a new job, or flaunting your assets to increase your finances, our pursuit for perfection can easily turn into an unhealthy obsession. 'SEX, DRUGS & PROTEIN SHAKES: The Pursuit of the Perfect Body' explores, unravels and explains the experiences of three young men as they share their compelling personal struggles, pleasures, joys and anxieties while they attempt to create the perfect physique.

Join me, Joseph Shield, as I present these young men's insightful, raw and gripping life stories.

Best wishes,

Joseph Shield

# CHAPTER ONE

# In Pursuit of the Perfect Body

Not so long ago, a twenty two-year-old male from Sydney, Australia was found unconscious in a sauna whilst on holiday in Bangkok, Thailand. "Zyzz", a well-known amateur bodybuilder with a cult following on YouTube and Facebook, had died from a heart attack. Soon after, his brother was arrested and pleaded guilty to the possession of anabolic steroids. Mass media attention followed, telling the story of a once "skinny kid" who transformed his body into a muscled Adonis through weight lifting, strict nutritional habits and alleged use of steroids. In an interview with an American bodybuilding website 'Zyzz' discusses his motivation for cultivating the ideal muscular male physique.

*"...I was always an extreme ectomorph. I could eat anything and not put on fat, muscle, or weight, or so I thought. I was always fascinated with bodybuilding but lacked the motivation to start training hard until after...my final year of school – it was time for a lifestyle change. I was ridiculously thin, the skinniest guy in my grade in school; people always commented on how skinny I was and I hated it... I remember feeling like a little bitch when I was out with girls, walking next to them and feeling the same size as them...I started going clubbing every weekend and always noticed whenever a jacked [muscular] dude walked by, they had a presence a lot greater than that of a 'normal' person. The guys respect them, and the girls are all over them, and really, who wouldn't want that?...Originally, it started out innocently enough, I wanted to get bigger so I wasn't so skinny, and have a bit of a build on me to impress girls. I'd look at pictures of*

*shredded guys and tell myself, that's going to be me. 4 years into my training, I can safely say that my motivation to train goes far beyond that of merely impressing people, it is derived from the feeling of having set goals and achieving the...My end goal is not to be some massed up freak, but rather to have a physique that can be looked as art; streamlined, tapered, and universally appealing."*

'Zyzz's explanation of his motivation for cultivating his body from an object that evoked personal disapproval to a desirable object of art makes you think – when does a perceived healthy lifestyle of exercise and nutrition become detrimental to one's health and well-being?

Whilst this desire for many young men like Zyzz to transform their bodies, sometimes at any cost, to become more aesthetically pleasing is not a recent phenomena; it is a growing trend that is quickly becoming the norm for many young men throughout the world. 'The Sydney Morning Herald' proclaims that the young men of today have become "The Steroid Generation" in its article on young men and their bodily pursuit of excellence. American Psychiatrist Harrison Pope, who specializes in body image coined the term 'The Adonis Complex' to describe body image concerns of young men. He states: "these concerns range from minor annoyances to devastating and sometimes even life-threatening obsessions – from a manageable dissatisfaction to full blown psychiatric body image disorders." In one form or another, the Adonis Complex touches millions of boys and men and inevitably, the people in their lives." The excessive preoccupation with muscularity is identified as Muscle Dysmorphia (MDD) or 'Bigorexia', and consequently an individual's obsession with their body can interfere with their social, educational, or occupational functioning. Social research suggests that young men's body obsession has been on the rise since the early 1970s. Research shows that 15% of American men were dissatisfied with their bodies in 1972 compared to 43% in 1997. 'The National Survey for Young Australians' reports that body image was perceived to be the number one issue of 'concern/importance' for 32.3% of 29,000 adolescent boys, aged 11-24.

So why are so many young men concerned with the appearance of their bodies? Over the last ten to fifteen years the western world has seen the rise of the sexualised, semi-naked, muscular, masculine male physique - the 'aesthetic-athletic' body. The 'aesthetic-athletic' body has been increasingly portrayed in television, magazines, the internet, social media and advertising media. The sexualised and eroticized male body has become the norm, particularly within the worlds of fashion, sport, fitness and health. The association between the muscular eroticized male body and good health (and fitness) can be apprehended within any book store as rows of glossy magazines displaying masculine muscular male physiques, with titles like 'Men's Health and Fitness', 'Men's Health', 'Muscle and Fitness', are displayed prominently, informing the reader that this is what a healthy body looks like. Many young men have swarmed to this imagery and ideology like bees to honey. 'Men's Health' circulation has sky rocketed from 250,000 to over 1.5 million in less than a decade and public exposure to the male form within glamour and cosmopolitan magazines has shown a dramatic rise in the percentage of semi naked male models, increasing from as little as 3% in the late 1950s to 36% by 1998. Similar trends have been found on American television with a 407% increase in nudity on prime time television since 2012.

The ideal 'aesthetic-athletic' male body represented within the media exhibits characteristics of a strong, muscular, attractive, successful, wealthy, happy, popular man who has status and sex appeal. In contrast the skinny, large, short or feminine male body represents a weak, unhealthy, unsuccessful, unattractive, lazy, 'gay', inferior man with little status and certainly no sex appeal. This was evident in a recent Time Magazine cover where the image of a skinny male flexing his biceps to the title 'THE WIMPY RECOVERY' was used to symbolize the world's recovery from the 2008 recession. Whilst many have embraced and celebrated this opportunity to express themselves and their bodies freely to the rest of the world without fear or condemnation, it has also resulted in many young men becoming obsessed with their bodies to the point where they feel anxious, depressed, physically inadequate and dissatisfied.

Throughout my childhood I had a love of action and comic heroes, WWF Wrestling and sport, but it never occurred to me that I would want to look like these characters. Even so, I was impressed by their athletic and muscular bodies and ascribed to what they represented - strong, masculine, tough, fit, skilful, attractive, popular, successful, super-human males. I would re-enact scenarios with my GI Joe, He-man, teenage mutant ninja turtles and WWF Wrestlers figurines, shaping my thoughts on what I perceived to be masculine identities, and perhaps unknowingly shaping my thoughts about my own body. My perceptions of a masculine male body, gained through playing with my figurines would have been different if I had been playing with the same figurines 30 years earlier or even today. Research into the bodies of popular boy's toys like the G.I. Joe shows a 'mesomorphic' transformation since the 1960's. In 1964 G.I. Joes had biceps with measurements equivalent to 12 inches on the male body; by 1974 15 inch biceps had developed with visible abdominals, by 1991 they had 16.5 inch biceps with additional 6-pack abdominals and a reduced waist creating the desirable 'V' shaped back and torso, and by the mid-1990's the 'G.I. Joe Extreme' figurine had pumped himself up to enormous 27 inch biceps. The evolution of the G.I. Joe figurine demonstrates how a child's perception and expectations of the male body may have changed over time. American Natural body builder and fitness model Sadik Hadzovic shares how his childhood was shaped by comic books and action figures:

> *"I always have been fascinated by the physiques in comic books and action figures that I played with as a child. Since a young age I knew how I wanted to look like and I wanted to resemble those action figures, comic book characters, and superheroes. I would always do hundreds of dumbbell curls and push-ups as a kid..."*

From a young age I was diagnosed with hyperlipidemia, high cholesterol, which had been passed down genetically through my family. I was encouraged by the medical specialists to live a healthy lifestyle and to maintain a healthy body by participating regularly in physical activity and by eating a low fat diet. I was monitored with annual blood tests and body examinations to ensure that everything was in order. The need for constant monitoring, medical surveillance and regulation of my body through my own eyes and those of the medical specialists has always been a part of my life. The need for constant maintenance of one's body and health is further reinforced through the attitudes and expectations of family and friends, the mass media, popular culture, schools and government surveillance. In recent times government health promotion campaigns, via the television and print media, have highlighted an apparent obesity epidemic. Health, or fear, campaigns illustrate the pitfalls of failing to keep your body in check. If 'YOU' do not control your weight through regular physical activity and a healthy diet you will suffer from increased tiredness, potential heart disease, and you will not be physically capable of looking after your children, as highlighted by various health campaigns throughout the world (e.g. 'push play', 'jump rope for heart' and 'measure up'). Emphasis is placed on the individual to take care of his or her own health and well-being. In Australia, and many other parts of the world, individuals are encouraged to sign up for private health insurance by receiving tax reductions, reinforcing the need for individual responsibility and reducing the state government's accountability for health and well-being. I have seen the consequences of this first hand as a health educator, where individuals try to take their personal health into their own hands. I have seen students and friends resorting to high risk and quick fix solutions for weight loss, such as excess exercising, potentially harmful 'fad' diets and eating practices, drugs, expensive supplements, creams and lotions or even cosmetic surgery in order to avoid being labelled as someone with 'poor' health who exhibits an unhealthy body. A YMCA study in the United Kingdom surveying 810 young men between the ages of 11 and 16 found that a third of them (270), said that they would resort to cosmetic surgery in order to achieve 'healthy', 'muscular', 'ideal' bodies so that they could embody the physiques of their favourite television stars. A trend that has been documented by a range of reality television shows: "Let Me In", "Extreme Makeover", "I Want a Famous Face" and "The Swan".

Health promotion, body surveillance and individual responsibility were key aspects of health and well-being within the education system as I progressed through High School. Being physically active and a very 'sporty' teenager I escaped the feelings of rejection and embarrassment that many others felt because I had an accepted 'healthy' body. Those that did not meet the criteria of a 'healthy' or socially accepted body were often teased, made fun of and were often deemed physically inferior because they were smaller, larger, less masculine or physically less capable. 'Normative' body types were reinforced during Physical Education lessons where students were measured, weighed, timed and recorded during fitness and health lessons and compared to national norms and regulated as 'normal', 'high ability', 'low ability' or 'poor'. Being physically fit and active I was usually ranked highly and received positive feedback that validated my physical skills and acceptable body, but I wonder how other students viewed their bodies after being labelled as 'low ability' or physically 'poor'? These students were probably left feeling physically deficient, embarrassed, self-conscious and 'down' because they did not meet the criteria for a socially accepted physical body.

After my university years I began my career in education as a secondary teacher in London, England. I had always been physically active and enjoyed sport, playing at representative level, so I decided to join a gym to stay physically active. Initially I was slightly intimidated by the more muscular tanned bodies displayed in synchronised gym attire that revealed their well-sculpted bodies. Before too long the gym had become a second home where I would exercise religiously five days a week. After all, who could resist the heated pools, Jacuzzi, saunas, and the attractive 'scenery' to escape the miserable grey days in old London town. I enjoyed the gym environment. Not only was it a place to exercise, but a place to socialise with newly made friends, and relax and unwind after a stressful day's work in the classroom.

After three years of working in London, I decided to move to sunnier shores in Sydney, Australia. I lived in the Eastern Suburbs, close to the beautiful beaches that aligned the shore. With long hot summer days and mild winters, it's not long before you realise that having a desirable beach body is essential. Surrounded by guys with loose fitting tank tops, who proudly display their hard-worked sculptured bodies on the beaches and streets of Sydney, it's not surprising that one starts to feel self-conscious about one's own body. This heightened bodily awareness is reinforced by the number of health and cosmetic-enhancing businesses that line the streets: tanning, waxing and beauty salons, cosmetic surgeries including hair implants, fat reduction, face lifts and the pre-summer essential botox injection, an array of health and wellness professionals, nutritional supplement stores, and of course, fitness centres where personal trainers eagerly promise to turn your flab into fabulous muscle.

Throughout my teaching career, my students - adolescents between the ages of 15 and 18 - have told me about their dreams of being famous, rich and living the 'high life'. The 'high life' represents having a high status so that you can get what you want - fast cars, sexy girls, and wicked parties, all attained through having good looks, a good body, and a good job, which usually equates to being a musician, a sports star or an actor. However, the need to develop skills and knowledge in order to achieve success, which may include fame and fortune, is usually not part of their plans, as they believe that good fortune will make it happen. And who can blame them? Reality television shows like 'Jersey Shore' and 'Keeping Up with the Kardashians' portray groups of young good looking men and women with no apparent skills or talent, other than strutting and parading their well-groomed and desirable bodies as they go from party to party living the perceived good life. These shows reinforce the idea that all you need in life to succeed is to embody physical perfection.

It is therefore no surprise that I had male teenagers often asking me about steroids and image-enhancing drugs to attain a more desirable masculine muscular physique. The young 'Aussie' men I taught were usually influenced by the rugby league, beach and 'Aussie' male bravado cultures that surrounded them. Strong, masculine, athletic, muscular professional athletes would take to the field on prime time television every Thursday to Monday, during the 'footy' season. Demonstrating their skills and well trained athletic physiques, displaying well inked arms, torsos and thighs, wrapped in short shorts, tight fitting aerodynamic football tops, and the occasional bloodied head bandage, revealing every muscular movement as they take to battle every week. In an effort to mimic the bodies of their heroes, students would often debate amongst themselves how they would achieve a more desirable body, and some had already started. Discussions ranged from different diet strategies, weight training programmes – heavy verse light weights, high or low repetitions, to steroids versus human growth hormones and so on.

Achieving the 'aesthetic-athletic' body without engaging in the rigorous daily regimes of professional athletes is most likely an unachievable mission for most young men, especially when they are at an age when their bodies are still developing physically. A minority of young men will develop a muscular mesomorphic physique in their teenage years, but the majority of them will be the everyday 'lanky' teenager that you see in the school playgrounds. Therefore, the 'ideal' body becomes unattainable, and young men around the age of twenty begin to look for alternatives and sources of hope, like sports supplements or steroids, to achieve their desired body.

The death of 'Zyzz' has put the spotlight on men's bodily practices and grabbed the attention of the Australian media and its audience, with an ever-increasing concern for young men's health and well-being.

A sub-culture of young men is placing an emphasis on getting bigger at all costs, and experts warn that the problem is affecting more young men than was previously thought. Image-enhancing drugs are becoming the norm, potentially placing the lives of young men at risk. Common drugs taken to improve physical appearance include: Clenbuterol ('Clen'), Anabolic steroids (Sustagen, Deca-Durabolin or Trenabol), Human Growth Hormones (HGH) and the tanning drug Malanotan, all of which can cause seriously detrimental side effects ranging from depression and insomnia to cardiovascular failure and cancer of the liver.

Performance and image-enhancing drugs, in my experience are predominantly sold and purchased 'underground' through word of mouth, on the street, within fitness centres, through personal trainers or gym members who sell it on behalf of their dealers, and even online via the internet. The amount of steroids being smuggled into Australia has more than doubled in the past five years. In the year 2011, Australian Customs made 2695 seizures of steroids and human growth hormones (HGH), a 155 percent increase on the 1054 seizures made between 2004 and 2005. These body-altering substances can come at a cost, as individuals will pay large amounts of money to achieve the perfect body they so desperately want to achieve, with a 'cycle' (duration of time) of steroids or HGH costing anything from $500 - $5000 dollars. However, un-prescribed and unregulated drugs are not always what they seem! Whilst living in Sydney a friend of mine bought a 'cycle' of HGH at the cost of approximately $5000 dollars via the internet. After the purchase had been made and the HGH had been delivered, upon inspection my friend became suspicious and decided to get them independently tested. Scientific testing showed that the liquid inside the vials was H2O/water. An expensive lesson in vanity had been learnt. Young men in the United States have also reported stories of supposed vials of anabolic steroids containing vinegar, olive oil, gasoline, sugar and salt solutions, rat poison or a customised alcohol solution. Whilst most have lived through this ordeal, there are many who haven't.

The desire to cultivate an individualised, masculine, 'aesthetic-athletic' body and an identity associated with status, personal success, and to be sexually attractive and desirable to others is an issue that needs to be addressed within youth sub-cultures not only within Australia, but throughout the world. This book explores how young men's body image affects their every day lives and experiences, and attempts to answer the following questions. How do young men consciously use their bodies as a canvas to develop and construct their physical appearance in order to achieve the 'aesthetic-athletic' body? What do young men perceive that they will achieve in changing their physical appearance and what influences them to do so? Where does this desire to attain the 'ideal body' come from? Does the process of working towards the ideal male body type change their every day experiences, and has their changing body enabled them to achieve the outcomes and desires they were searching for as a young man in contemporary society? And has the search for the desired ideal male body been detrimental and/or beneficial to their health and well-being?

# THREE YOUNG MEN

Rocco, Jack and Joe are three young Australian men in their mid twenties who live and work in the multi-cultural metropolitan city of Sydney; a city known for it's temperate climate, beautiful beaches, sexy bodies, laid back locals, and outdoor lifestyle.

Rocco is a 25-year-old middle-class Anglo-saxon male who has established a career in advertising. He enjoys fine dining, fast cars and living the good life.

Jack is a 24-year-old middle-class male of mixed race who is employed as a pharmaceutical sales manager. He enjoys playing sport, travelling and relaxing at home.

Joe is a 24-year-old working-class Anglo-saxon male who is a social worker offering support for young men who have criminal histories. He enjoys bodybuilding, watching television, listening to popular music and spending quiet nights in on the sofa.

The following three chapters focus on the lives of these three young Australian men, exploring and analysing the ways in which they experience their body image within in a city that values good looks and well tanned muscular physiques.

# CHAPTER TWO

# Critical Moments

## Puberty, Acne and Sexual Desire

Early adolescence and puberty emerged as a crucial time in the young men's lives for reflecting upon their own and others' (school peers) body image and appearance. In response to the question – "when did you start to reflect upon the appearance of your body?" the young men predominantly identified puberty as a pivotal 'critical moment':

*"When I was 13-14…Junior high school, when I started to be attracted to girls I became aware of what physical attributes they liked in guys…I was single and couldn't get any dates. [I felt] unwanted and left out. [I] decided to start taking care of my body and getting in shape." (Rocco)*

*"umm…puberty I guess. Noticing attractive guys…wanting to look similar to the ones I thought were good looking…that's probably when I got serious about it…thinking about how I look…I was border line obese. 90kg. So not good…I felt fat and ugly. I also had really bad acne. Not attractive and lacked a lot of confidence." (Jack)*

*14. When I was in high school….and I saw a rugby player with big quads and I was like oh I want mine like that. I was ugly, I was skinny.….acne…I went from being a very pretty boy to an acne riddled reject…I looked at myself and thought wow I have nothing goin' for me…other than great hair." (Joe)*

These statements support notions advanced by developmental theorists and psychologists such as Erik Erikson (1902-1994), Jean Piaget (1896-1980) and Urie Bronfenbrenner (1917- 2005), who suggest that adolescence is a critical time when young people shape their bodily dispositions and practices. According to these theorists, adolescence is characterised by physiological, neurological and psychological changes prompted by increases in hormone production. Anecdotal evidence also supports the changes associated during adolescence, for example when I was working as a secondary school teacher, teachers would talk about the 'silly (mating) season' during spring. They referred to this season as a time when young adolescent boys and girls would seemingly be hysterical with each other, chasing each other in the school grounds, continuously flirting and displaying instances of affection. Examples of such tales of 'hysteria' where adolescents have been infatuated with each other due to increased levels of hormones have been documented throughout history. American sexuality researchers Komisaruk, Beyer-Flores & Whipple state:

> *"From ancient Greece to Freud's time, doctors stimulated orgasms in women via "medical massage" to treat the catchall female ailment known as hysteria. In the late 1800s, the vibrator was designed for the same purpose."*

The enduring regularity with which this tale has been told throughout history would lead one to assume that puberty is a natural adolescent phase, generating significant changes in young men's, and women's, bodily appearance and experiencing their bodies in a phenomenological sense. For better or for worse, Joe, Jack and Rocco noticed changes which included a heightened sense of self-consciousness, increased hair growth and body odour, a deepening of the voice, increased testosterone levels, increased sexual attraction to others, the physiological ability to procreate with others, and of course, acne. These physiological and psychological changes appeared to have had a profound affect on the way they viewed and experienced their own bodies and interacted with others. The young men described how they felt "fat and ugly", "skinny" and "rejected" within their social networks. This would suggest that their embodied undesirable physical changes were perceived to be symbolic of ugliness, which was deemed to affect negatively their social capital, power and status amongst their school peers. Therefore they considered themselves unlikely to attain a "mate" despite their hormones apparently suggesting that now would be a good time to find one.

Is this perceived apparent 'mating season' behaviour and excitement purely developmental or is it a tale whereby myth has bred 'reality'? Is it assumed that all young men and women need help to relieve themselves of 'hysteria' or is this phenomenon simply socially constructed? Are increased levels of physiological arousal restricted to adolescence or are they simply restrained and controlled as we grow into adulthood through societal pressures in order to behave in ways that are deemed as socially acceptable? And is there really such a thing as heightened sexual desire during particular seasons of the year?

To compound these young men's issues associated with the physiological changes occurring within their bodies they were also expected to meet various social norms (e.g. the need to look good), via the surveillance and expectations of their friends, family and popular culture, who reinforced the undesirability of "ugliness". The pressures to meet social bodily norms are evident in Rocco's, Jack's and Joe's testimonies. For example, during the process of recalling their first memories whereby they consciously thought about and reflected back upon their bodies and identities, they remember comparing their perceived undesirable young bodies to the more popular, muscular and attractive guys (e.g. the rugby player who showcased muscular quadriceps) within their social environment. Consequently, as these young men observed and compared their perceived under-developed muscles and beauty, comparatively speaking, they experienced feelings of decreased confidence, low-self esteem and diminished self-worth. Therefore, Joe, Jack and Rocco - who did not obtain these desirable physical traits - often condemned their own bodies as they felt the social pressure to aspire to and construct a more desirable physique that is symbolic of sex appeal. Re-constructing their bodies to attain physical capital and the attention and acceptance of others, was regarded as a possible strategy that might improve their social capital. This would enable them to manipulate and acquire power and status within their social environments, and in their eyes, attract others and "get dates".

Friends and peers within the social worlds of these young men exacerbated the anguish and anxiety which resulted from displaying an unattractive bodily appearance. Rocco states:

> *"[There was] peer pressure to have a GF [girl-friend] in school. The need came from being a teenager and wanting to fit in."*

In Rocco's case, finding a girlfriend was perceived as an important part of being an adolescent, increasing his social capital and ensuring acceptance amongst his peers. This objective was perceived as unattainable on account of his skinny, ugly, acne-riddled body, as indicated by his comment: "I was single and couldn't get any dates. [I felt] unwanted and left out." These experiences of feeling unpopular, unwanted, embarrassed and alone left Rocco and the other young men to transition from the process of reflecting upon and surveilling their bodies through the more desirable and popular bodies of others in their early adolescence (ages 13 to 14) to constructing bodies that would help them to attract others and enable more social acceptance in their mid adolescence (ages 16 to 19).

All three young men experienced feelings of 'ugliness' because their existing adolescent bodies did not reflect the physical beauty of the male mesomorphic (muscular) physique often identified by young men as the ideal body. That is, an 'aesthetic-athletic' body that people frequently associate with positive stereotypes, including happy, polite, helpful, brave, strong, masculine, healthy, self-reliant, and smart. In contrast, endomorphic (fat) (and acne-covered bodies) are perceived and experienced as ugly, lazy, unwanted, lonely, unattractive and less intelligent. These common stereotypes are often socially constructed through various discourses (health, beauty and success) within popular culture and mass media, which inform and shape our conscious and unconscious minds as to how we should experience our bodies when we display a particular body image. These phenomenological experiences have been documented throughout Western cultures, with sociological and psychological research suggesting strong cultural preferences toward a mesomorphic, muscular, male body and an aversion towards endomorphic (fat) and ectomorphic (skinny) male bodies.

However, the perceptions and experiences associated with a fat body have not always been interpreted and experienced as a negative state of being. American Historian P. Stearns states:

> "Between the 1860's and the 1880's, rotundity gained ground for men as well as women...Doctors urged the importance of solid weight in their growing campaign against nervousness. A decent belly on a man denoted prosperity and sensible good health. A little paunch above the belt was something to be proud of. Even as some interest emerged in Europe amid medical advice concerning moderation, Americans persisted in maintaining their full-figure standards throughout he 1880's and beyond. .... Interest in exercise did begin to increase for both men and women, but it was not initially associated with slenderness and muscularity."

These insights into societal perceptions, historically and from the perspectives of Joe, Rocco and Jack suggest that the way in which many young men interpret and experience the shape and appearance of their bodies is linked to the social discourses, attitudes and expectations that surround them at the time. These discourses are reinforced through the popular culture, word of mouth and the constant surveillance of friends, family, teachers, doctors and politicians within the socio-cultural spaces that they live. They may and often do, change over time.

## Muscles, Sexuality and Porn Stars

Afer the initial transitional period of puberty to adulthood, a time of observation, self-awareness and reflection of one's physical self through the perceived attractive bodies of others, these young men progressed to the next stage. During mid adolescence, between the ages of 16 to 19, Jack, Rocco and Joe deliberately constructed 'ideal' individual bodies and identities. Their identities have seemingly been influenced by the unique experiences and interpretations of the various discourses and social messages that surround them within the various social communities they live. In response to the question: "When did you purposefully decide to construct the appearance of your body?" Joe responded:

> "I didn't start working out till I was 16 and I did it just cos [because] I wanted to be big... not for anyone else...there was a switch and BOOM...the only time a person or image influenced my behaviour in the way I saw and perceived my body...was when I saw a porno in America...I looked at this porn star and thought yup that's what I'm goin' too look like...I was 19. I wanted to reach his physical level...I wanted big legs... big booty...I didn't care what others wanted or suggested how I look...people saying I'm fine the way I am.....I didn't care. I idolized him...I wanted to wear shorts and have...smooth bulgin' legs. It appealed to me...I like who I was.....I did then and do now...it wasn't about oh I need that and want it then oh I will be more attractive...it was a goal I wanted...just for personal gratification."

Throughout the interview Joe stresses the point that the body construction behaviours and practices he engaged in to become "big" [muscular] were adhered to strictly for intrinsic reasons. He enjoyed the process of constructing and achieving a more muscular physique. BOOM! He enjoyed the experience of watching his physique change and found it personally gratifying to work on his body. He testifies that he did not attempt to change his body in order to acquire physical, cultural or symbolic capital, neither was it to please others, to gain attention or to create a more desirable identity. He simply enjoyed the process of watching his body develop. Joe's ambition to become more muscular would appear to be influenced by the various discourses of muscularity, masculinity, beauty and attractiveness as exhibited by the American porn star he observed and modeled himself upon. However, these social messages, which perspire from Adonis-like porn stars, appear seemingly invisible to Joe as he is unaware of the reasons why he is fixated with their muscular bodies and why he perceives them as desirable. Pierre Bourdieu, an influential French sociologist, describes this process as 'doxa', whereby dominant social messages transmitted through the media on behalf of private business and governments inform an individuals' knowledge, practices and subjectivities regarding the ways that they should present themselves to the world and behave. These social messages become embedded within one's psyche, a "learned ignorance" that is accepted as natural. In other words, young men like Joe unknowingly become victims of the hidden agendas of private businesses who deliberately construct images that they portray as desirable and pleasurable in the hope that the public will buy their products.

These social messages appear to have had a significant impact on the ways that many young men like Joe, Jack and Rocco make sense of their bodies. From a phenomenological perspective, they inform the various benefits that Joe perceives he will experience from constructing a muscular taut body that he and others can admire and as an attractive, evolving art form in which he can be proud of. His visions of a transformative, (in a physical and psychological sense), muscular body seemingly provided him with physical capital - increased muscle mass - that he could exhibit to himself, the mirror and others by wearing more revealing shorts that showcased his big booty and smooth bulgin' legs. This new self that he wanted to create was a far cry from the acne-riddled reject he embodied.

In response to the same question, Jack responded:

*"Initially in Uni when I was really fat that I decided to lose the weight...At Uni it was getting physically uncomfortable being fat...It felt really good getting into shape. Whatever the reason was for these critical moments the positive effect on my health were definitely a great advantage and soon the reason to continue change...for physical well-being. I guess also that in a way watching porn...everyone had perfect bodies and I guess that would also be a reason to want a better body. And when you see other guys with attractive body types and you don't have one yourself it makes you want to change it."*

Jack's initial reason for reconstructing his body was to lose weight, as he started to become physically uncomfortable carrying excess weight (fat).

*"When I ran my stomach [abdomen] and back fat would jiggle... was a struggle with a little bit of exercise. Just felt gross and lethargic. My thighs would constantly chaff."*

Once Jack started to loose his body fat the improved sense of health and physical well-being he experienced increased his motivation to continue with his body constructing practices. Like Joe, initially he seemed to be unaware of the social influences that caused him to reshape his body through weight training and trying to eat healthier, but he nevertheless felt healthier for doing so. This brings me to the question: Are feelings of good health perceived - from a phenomenological viewpoint - psychologically induced via the socially constructed health messages that invade young men's daily lives or are they purely physiologically induced? For instance, the increased ability of a person's lungs to inhale, exhale and diffuse oxygen to red blood cells throughout the body, which improves one's ability to breathe more effectively and to develop stronger muscles as a result of cardio-vascular exercise. Jack's perception of bodily good health or of feeling "gross" is understood through his interpretations of the knowledge within his social surroundings. These young men's various experiences of their bodies, contradictory and complex as they are, could therefore also be argued to be psychosomatic, whereby they perceive pleasurable (or unpleasant) feelings from the phenomena of good health, therefore, it occurs. For example, whilst Jack complained of chaffing from carrying excess fat, other acquaintances have told me of the chaffing that they have incurred on their legs and stretch marks around the pectoral and shoulder muscles from developing excess muscle, due to weight training. However, these bodily occurrences were not perceived as a signal of poor health. They were perceived as a positive side effect of sculpting the ideal body. I would suggest that these contrasting states of mind, of that which is perceived as healthy, are influenced by the social ideals (e.g. that a fat body is unhealthy) that individuals are familiar with within their social environments. Therefore, one's psycho-physiological bodily experiences, i.e. feeling healthy and energetic or fat and gross, can be induced by the way that young men perceive the socially constructed messages surrounding them which often inform the men of the need to measure and shape up to bodily ideals, i.e. a body that is taught, athletic and well groomed.

Upon greater reflection Jack acknowledges that watching pornography and other idealised attractive images of other male bodies within his own social fields may have influenced his behaviour on a subconscious level. Consequently, these 'ideal' male bodies provide a blueprint of what is perceived to be socially desirable, attractive and wanted by many young men like Jack, Joe and Rocco. Furthermore, Rocco, reflects upon the reasons why he felt the need to construct a more desirable body:

*"...when I left school and realized I was gay, image and "looks" became very important to get attention, make friends and be desired – this is when I started to work on my physique."*

The realisation and exploration of a person's sexual identity is a common occurrence during adolescence. This transition, realisation and understanding of a person's sexuality seems to play a significant role in how young men's body image, identity and bodily constructing practices are shaped. Discourses of competition emerge from Rocco's statement as he feels the need to reconstruct his body into a more socially desirable version of himself in order to compete successfully with others which will enable him to receive attention, make friends and find a date. In order to gain acceptance within this community Rocco consciously started to reconstruct his physical body and 'look', using his physical capital, to get the attention he was seeking from other young gay men. Acquiring social status and power within Rocco's social spaces, via the use of a reconstructed desirable body, is perceived by Rocco as being crucial for establishing successful friendships and relationships within the gay community he interacts with.

A person's bodily appearance and practices seem to influence the way in which their sexuality and sexual desire is expressed towards others. This was observed over a six-month period as I noticed the behaviour of a young student at a university gym. This young man had been training regularly with a friend for the first four months of the university calendar year. However, one day the situation had suddenly changed. This young man had suddenly exchanged his loyal training partner for a potential girlfriend, and in doing so appeared as a more well-groomed version of his former self. There was a new hair cut, a tidier appearance, a permanent smile entrenched on his face, a proud strut and happy skip in his step as he appeared to float around the university gym on 'cloud nine' (a happy habitual space). Meanwhile his former training partner was left to train by himself. When a male suddenly finds an attractive mate it would appear he will do all that he can to maintain the relationship. It's often not until he finally says; "I do" that the extra kilograms of fat start to pile on again.

## Time to Get Serious

As these young men progressed through adolescence, from high school to university and into the workforce, and strived to make more meaningful relationships with others, the importance they placed upon their bodily appearance increased. Jack, John and Rocco increased the intensity of their body constructing practices in an attempt to significantly increase their physical and social capital by creating a body and identity that was perceived to be more desirable to them and others. Jack made the following comment in regards to the critical moments in his life when he purposefully started to reconstruct his physical appearance:

> "...it wasn't till I got to Sydney that I started to radically change my body. When I moved here the gym gave me something to do after work but it was also driven by the expectation of body image...In Sydney it was expectations in a way of body image and...well...as improving my body for improving confidence."

Jack describes how living in a different social space, having moved from New Zealand to Sydney triggered the need for him to radically reconstruct his body image. This shift yielded a significant effect on his perception of his own body, which was subjected to increased scrutiny, surveillance and social expectations from those that surrounded him in the new environment he now lived in. In Sydney he felt he had to radically construct a new body and identity, taking on a more attractive physique and appearance so that he would feel more socially accepted by others. Jack's comment conveys the importance of the social spaces in which one lives and how one social environment can shape and influence an individuals' bodily appearance, identity and their sense of who they are – accepted, unwanted, desirable or unattractive. Whether a person lives in uptown Manhattan, New York, a farm ranch in Dallas, Texas, inside a mosque in Dubai or in Sydney, Australia surrounded by surf, sand and Speedos, the environment's unique cultures, landscapes and history arguably influence one's perception of what is and what is not a desirable and acceptable body and identity. In order for one to acquire social acceptance and power within a social space, the use of one's physical capital is often vital. In Jack's process of shaping up and "improving" his body in order to meet the social norms of his new living space, he reports feelings of increased confidence as he begins to feel more comfortable within his own body and to feel increasingly accepted within his new habitat.

The varying social environments that these young men interacted and socialised within also provided critical moments within these young men's lives, which seem to have influenced the way in which they perceived their bodies and their desire or need to reconstruct their physical appearance and identity. Rocco states:

*"Body image was very important when I started working... because I worked in a tanning salon! Face and clothes became important when I started my corporate jobs...I got a PT. He taught me about nutrition and training. In hindsight, he probably wasn't actually that good, but he definitely got me started!"*

Once Rocco entered the workforce and began to work within the corporate world he started to place a greater emphasis on his appearance. Rocco recognised the importance of constructing a body that would enable him to acquire physical, symbolic and economic capital. A body that would be perceived by himself, his employer and his customers as consumer-friendly in order to ensure that he could sell a particular product (e.g. beauty). Consequently his bodily appearance had become a valuable asset that he could use to his advantage to make a living. Sociology scholars Patterson and Elliot state:

*"Indeed, as consumer society evolves, and people are defined less and less by their work roles, identity projects are increasingly tied to the internalization of commodities through consumption. As a result of commodification, bodies are ascribed exchange-value,*

*that is, they seem to possess physical capital...Within particular*
*social fields, bodily attributes, such as aesthetic qualities, are*
*ascribed certain value and function as capital, which may*
*be subsequently converted to economic, cultural and social*
*capital. Moreover, this value increases, the closer those bodies*
*approximate to a social field's normalized ideals. Thus, men and*
*women are persuaded to devote their energies to improving their*
*bodies, thereby maximizing their exchange value and "we can*
*begin to see how bodily attributes function as currency, securing*
*further rewards and serving as a valuable resource". Such*
*commodification is supported by the body-maintenance industry*
*where youth, beauty, health and fitness become sources of physical*
*capital."*

Increasing numbers of young men, like Rocco, feel the need
to treat their bodies as a project whereby they re-invent, re-design,
package and brand themselves into valuable commodities in order to
compete against other employees, to attain and maintain a job and
income, and to gain an identity that their employers can use to their full
advantage in order to acquire business. In contemporary times one's
body and identity, influenced by the profusion of social messages from
popular culture that often inform the bodily practices they engage in
and the appearance they create, are encouraged to portray socially
constructed desirable characteristics which are perceived to be valuable
assets within the corporate world. A physical schema that embodies
a well-groomed 'aesthetic-athletic' beauty is regularly perceived to
demonstrate personal attributes of good health, intelligence, trust,
honesty, desirability, success and machine like efficiency with an
ability to get things done. American social commentator Andrew
Kimbrell suggests:

*"Our association of the body with 'efficient machines' has crept*
*into our culture. It has created a modern body type in the*
*machine's image...[the] 'techno-body'. The techno-body ideal, for*
*men, and increasingly for women, is the 'lean, mean machine':*

*a hairless, overly muscled body, occasionally oiled, which very much resembles a machine."*

Therefore, our bodies have become a machine-like organism that can be physically and mentally trained, constructed, altered, tailored and fixed, ready for the demands and rigoors of the 9-6 corporate life. The 'aesthetic-athletic' body, which is perceived as the embodiment of a healthy, attractive and efficient body - and, therefore a healthy intelligent mind - is often perceived as a healthy investment for many employers. However, for those who are unable to attain such a socially desirable physique their "exchange value" is considered to be of a significantly lower value. Consequently, Rocco's realisation of the importance of obtaining physical capital led him to consciously reflect upon his existing skinny body and commence the use of body re-constructing practices in order to transform his physical appearance into one that he considered to be socially desirable for the corporate world. Consequently, by constructing and embodying an attractive 'corporate' identity he now had the potential to acquire status, power and success within the fields that he worked and socialised. Manipulating these social spaces through the use of his body also allowed him to acquire economic (money) and social capital (increased popularity) by presenting an image that was embraced within the culture that he worked.

Furthermore, Rocco goes on to say:

*"I didn't feel much pressure to look good when I was dating girls. Guys were totally different. My first BFs [boyfriend's] were very attractive and I felt tremendous pressure to look good."*

Rocco recalls the pressure he felt when he began to date other young men and the critical role that his sexuality played in the way he thought about his body. The "tremendous pressure" he experienced to look good in order to allure other young men and to maintain a relationship was influential in his decision to construct and maintain an attractive physique and identity. This tremendous pressure to 'look good' was perceived to be of greater significance within the social domains of the gay community. It would seem - to Rocco at least - that the gay community places a greater emphasis on looks and physical attraction in order to attract and maintain meaningful relationships, especially when compared to the 'straight' community. American sociologist Jason Whitesel states:

> *"Like heterosexual women, gay men experience greater conflict with their appearance, physique and food when compared to heterosexual men, in part because gay men recognise the images everyone encounters of the idealised male body as being gay. Further, gay men negatively associate fat with effeminacy."*

Furthermore, the skinny body within the gay community is still seen - consciously and subconsciously - by many as symbolic of the HIV/AIDS era during the 1980s. Therefore, Rocco's first relationships with other young gay men plausibly had a profound affect on his own, and other gay men's, expectations of how his body should look, behave and interact with others. Rocco's capacity to construct a sexually appealing physique was perceived by him to be vital in manipulating his status and power within the gay community by acquiring sexual capital in order to increase his chances of developing sexual relationships with others.

Joe's critical moment in late adolescence, aged 23, occurred when socialising within various social networks i.e. work, school, the gym, and with friends. Joe recalls the following:

> *"...when I was 23 people always told me oh your so pretty pity your so skinny and I thought to myself...oh really and then I had put on nearly 18kgs of muscle...I was 54 kgs when I was 19... and then at 23 I was like BOOM...so I thought to myself oh really? Well fuck them I'll show em and once I get too my goal they can all rot ...it was quite malicious at the time...I hated everyone and I never went out...I never drank...I just worked*

*out, worked and studied...I was like oh well you may look down*
*at me now but one day you will be like oh that's why...that's why*
*I worked out so much, that's why I had those protein shakes...*
*that's why I went to the gym so much...that's why I sacrificed*
*so much and I never looked at them as bitter I just didn't want*
*anything to do with them. I used their negativity as stepping*
*stones."*

Joe describes how people perceived him as skinny despite developing a more muscular build since he had started weight training earlier in his adolescence. Embodying a 'skinny' physique was seen as a negative physical characteristic for Joe to have. Joe recalls people's comments and behaviour towards him as being malicious. Consequently, he decided to use this judgment against him as motivation to focus on constructing a more muscular body then he currently had. This statement, whereby he seems to be creating a body that reflects social expectations and norms, contradicts earlier comments where he adamantly testifies that the purpose and motivation for constructing a bigger and muscular body was for his own personal gratification. This demonstrates how individual interpretations and memories can affect one's recall of events which in turn shape one's personal subjectivity; specifically, who and what they are and how they became the person they perceive themselves to be.

The social undesirability and surveillance of the skinny body (as with the endomorphic/fat body discussed previously), as encountered by Joe, is socially constructed through popular culture and mass media, which often suggests that the ectomorphic (skinny) body is an undesirable trait for a male to embody. Ectomorphic male bodies have often been associated with being quiet, nervous, sneaky, afraid, less masculine, feminine, weak and sickly. These stereotypes can be found among a variety of male populations, including lower and middle classes, blacks and whites, children, and adults both young and old. In this instance the socio-psychological cost for Joe of not fitting the masculine cultural and social ideal was for him to engage

in anti-social practices, whereby he isolated himself in an attempt
to construct a more muscular physique as a consequence of socially
rejection, in an effort to seek personal pay-back and redemption. This
experience evidently had a dramatic affect on the formation of his
identity and the way he engaged with and perceived the 'world' in
which he lived.

## BOOM!

Whilst Jack and Rocco had a series of events and
experiences throughout their adolescence that
navigated and shaped how they thought about their bodies
Joe experienced a single moment that had a significant effect
on the way that he perceived his appearance. As alluded to
in the previous statement, at the age of 23 he experienced a
sudden and striking realisation. BOOM! An epiphany had
occurred that inspired him to continue reconstructing a
bigger, muscular, masculine version of himself. When asked
to clarify what he meant by BOOM! in his last statement he
replied:

> *"Went for it. I hit a switch in my body and just boom. Never
> looked back. Just did it. BOOM - like an explosion. Just did
> it, straight away. Nothing stopping it or preventing it...an
> explosion of hard work and determination. BOOM as in just
> kept working. Instant drive. Instant direction. Knew what I
> wanted. Didn't care how long it took."*

A significant thought concerning his bodily appearance had
occurred; psychologists call this a leap in understanding. This
new insight occured after many years of reflecting upon his own
pre-existing fleshy, skinny body; gathering information from perceived
social norms and popular culture in order to transform his body and
identity into a muscular Adonis. Through the use of various reflexive
body techniques Joe had found a way to construct a more formidable

body, which had a significant effect on his individual body practices. The reflexive body techniques that he used included weight lifting, nutrition, the new discovery of steroids and an increased desire to succeed. This was a discovery triggered by a new and key piece of information and an increased depth of understanding accompanied with various prior pieces of knowledge (e.g. strict diet and exercise), which together increased his understanding and his ability to create the body he desired.

Furthermore, Joe, added:

> "It wasn't a BOOM here come steroids. It was a BOOM. Time to use your insecurities, fears and thoughts of other people into something I can use to grow. BOOM. The thought process was instant."

BOOM! Joe had found a way to channel his negative feelings towards others after years of being made to feel inadequate from the bullying and harassment of others due to his skinny frame. Steroids had simply become a means to an end, enabling him to create a body in which he would feel comfortable, to improve his confidence, to have a sense of purpose and achievement, and to silence his critics.

## Critical Omissions

When interpreting these young men's stories it was interesting to uncover the discourses that did not emerge as critical moments that may have shaped their individual bodily appearances and subjectivities. Interestingly enough, these young men did not recall any experiences regarding their childhood. This is a period of time where many young boys throughout the world are often exposed to toys and media that encourage and reinforce masculine stereotypes such as muscular action figures like GI Joes, Thundercats, and superheroes with phenomenal super human powers, or

television shows like WWE (World Wrestling Entertainment),
or the 'aesthic-athletic' bodies of sporting heroes like David
Beckham (football), Lebron James (Basketball) and Rafael
Nadal (Tennis). Various psychological research studies have
revealed that these popular culture figures and icons can affect
the way in which many young men perceive and experience
their bodies. However, despite Joe, Rocco and Jack seemingly
being unaware of or unable to recall critical moments from
their childhood, this does not mean that such moments
had not occurred. This was noticeable when I observed one
of the young men's online social media profiles, which had
numerous images of male and female cartoon characters
(e.g. He-man, X-Men, Dragon Ball Z, Marvel Super Heroes)
showcasing characteristics of masculinity, bravery, strength,
and fearlessness embodied within strong, large, muscular,
taut bodies. This suggests that he was engaged with popular
culture figures during his childhood within his social spheres,
which may have influenced his perceptions of masculinity
and the characteristics and body practices required for him
to be perceived as a desirable young man. One could argue
that this lack of awareness of engaging with ultra masculine
and muscular images is - in a sense - a form of hegemony
or doxa (as used by Bourdieu), a learnt ignorance. Cultural
messages transmitted through children's media arguably act
as gender identity training that may unknowingly influence
and construct a young person's knowledge, shaping their
habits and sense of self within the communities they are
engaged with. Discourses and social messages of masculinity
are often socially constructed and shaped by capitalist media
tycoons who are eager to sell an appealing brand and product
to its young target audience so that they can make a healthy
profit. And let's be honest, which young boy does not want to
grow up with super human strength and a desirable muscular
physique which he can use to overcome evil and become the
hero of the day?

Although the potential influence of popular culture during a boy's childhood did not surface within these young men's stories it did appear when I asked Alex, who is both a friend and a well-known Sydney based personal trainer about his body image. He stated:

*"I don't think anything specifically has had a specific effect on me in terms of my body image etc. I've generally always been naturally lean, even as a kid I had abs. It's a bit weird. [laugh]."*

However, after a couple of days' reflection he made the comment:

*"When I was 8 years old I received the Hulkamania Workout Set for Christmas. Man was I excited!…It led to me training in the lounge in my short shorts and head band and my sisters laughing at me constantly. Did it stop me? Nope, and I had abs as an 11 year old!…Plus this means I can claim to have been weight training for over 20 years."*

This comment highlights the importance of reflexivity, recall; reflecting on ones life. Initially Alex recalls always being lean and having abs as a child. "Yeah right!" I hear you thinking. However, upon greater reflection he remembers the critical moment and the significance that the popular wrestling icon, Hulk Hogan had on constructing a desirable physique. This suggests that the ability of individuals to recall information is necessarily subjective. Their views are based on their recall of knowledge at a certain point of time, which may change depending on what they can remember. This comment also reflects that individual experiences are completely unique, and despite Rocco, Joe and Jack not recalling critical moments during their childhood - even after several days' reflection - this does not mean that it might not occur in others, as described by Alex.

The absence of discourses which discern popular culture was not the only notable omission from these young men's childhoods. It was also interesting to note that there were no critical moments that related to them experiencing any forms of harassment and bullying that may have had an effect on the experience and perception of their bodies. There were undertones of harassment within Joe's testimony but he constantly reinforced the message that the construction of his body was for personal gratification and not as a result of the torment he received throughout his adolescence, despite obvious contradictions that have been pointed out in this chapter. Incidences of young men being harassed during their childhood revealed in other psychology and sociology research throughout the Western world suggest that this is the case for many males, young and old. Being too fat, too skinny, too black, too white, ugly or having physical or learning difficulties often renders young people susceptible to abuse, which can affect their self-esteem, their confidence and the way that they comprehend and understand their bodies. These experiences of childhood bullying often leave permanent 'mental' scars, which affect the way that they socialise with others and which also affect the view of their own place within the world that they live. These young men often grow up to identify themselves as being stupid, unattractive, unintelligent and incapable of having a successful life, thus affecting how they engage with their lives and the expectations they place upon themselves. These experiences and feelings are often reinforced through popular culture and through the media when many children absorb negative social messages about those that are not physically attractive (e.g. the TV programme Ugly Betty, the story of the ugly duckling and numerous cartoon shows throughout history).

The male adolescents taking part in this research experienced a myriad of issues that acted as critical moments in the production of their bodies, identities and lives. These young men navigated their way through physiological change, sexual desire, sexuality and socially constructed discourses of fatness, thinness, ugliness and beauty, health, the media, and capitalism to make sense of the relationships and experiences that they have with their bodies and identities.

# CHAPTER THREE

# Sex in the City

## Constructing The Sexually Seductive Body

The number one theme that emerged from these young
men's personal stories was their conscious desire to
reconstruct their bodies and identities, using a variety of
grooming and body practices. These various techniques were
often used to transform their "fat" or "skinny" bodies into
more sexually enticing 'aesthetic-athletic' physiques that
they thought would help them to attain sexual relations
with others, and to afford a sense of self-gratification. The
body-altering routines, practices and services that many
young men including Rocco, Jack and Joe engage in include:
weight training, personal trainers, restrictive diets, nutrition
supplements, steroids, body hair removal, teeth whitening,
botox, facial make up, sunbeds and spray tans, and wearing
clothes that reveal and showcase their taught bodies. For
example Rocco and Jack commented:

*"I used it [various body practices] to pick up guys [and] my
current boyfriend. Gay guys like nice faces and hard bodies...
so I work on both. I want people to think that I look good and
that the hard work in the gym, with my eating program and
[that my] healthy lifestyle pays off. [I] appeal more to others and
feel more confident...It is important for a man to look M&M
[muscular and masculine] because that is what most people find
attractive about a man." (Rocco)*

"Yeah definitely food and supplements...I do watch my diet...
especially now that summer is coming up and I need to take my shirt
off. I also take cutters and fat blockers when I'm trying to shred [loose
weight].....Straight men use their body to impress women and other
men to feel more powerful. Gay men display [their bodies] to get
other gay men to want to have sex with them...gay guys work out to
get a good body and because they realize other guys are looking for
something similar and as one of my mates puts it ...If you're gay, no
pecs, no sex...straight guys that spend a lot of time looking good are
doing it for self satisfaction and probably some level of insecurity...as
long as they look healthy girls don't really care for physical appearance
as much. Emotional attachment to them is more appealing...and they
tend to go more for the man's man." (Jack)

These two statements provide an insight into the various practices
that Jack and Rocco use and their perceptions of the reasons they
choose to use them. In this instance their desire to acquire a more
physically attractive body and appearance was driven by a concern
to accumulate physical capital, something that they could leverage to
their advantage within the various social environments they interacted
with. Boosting their physical capital through reconstructing their
bodies and subjectivities was considered to be an important step
towards acquiring sexual and social capital, as this would increase
the likelihood of manipulating their new found social status and
becoming more appealing and attractive to others.

The young men draw on several discourses as they discuss the
symbolic capital that their body practices create. Health, beauty
and dominant notions of what masculinity entails seem particularly
evident in their commentaries. Rocco, for example discusses the
significance of representing a body and identity that portrays an image
of a healthy, muscular and masculine body, an achievement to which
he attributes increased confidence, the capacity to pick up guys and to
snare his current good-looking boyfriend. Jack suggests that achieving
a muscular body is not as crucial for men within the heterosexual

community. He suggests that females are not as shallow as gay men; placing greater importance on partner commitment, a traditional 'macho' male masculinity, a 'man's man' and health. Interestingly, Jack's actions actually contradict his own insights since he seems to place a significant emphasis on looking good as he attempts to reconstruct his once obese body into not only a healthy looking body, but also a more muscular and masculine one. So why do these young men consider a healthy body to be synonymous with muscularity, athleticism, beauty and sex appeal? These various social discourses and messages seem to have threaded themselves throughout the social worlds of each of these young men. The young men's individual social environments, albeit in different ways, has had a significant impact on how they have interpreted the various forms of body knowledge that surrounds them. In other words, the information passed on through the media, the government, popular culture and through friends appears to have influenced and shaped their personal understandings, perceptions, practices and experiences of their bodies and identities.

This acquired knowledge appears to have produced emotions of fear, anxiety and the desire for Jack, Rocco and Joe in order to avoid exhibiting an unhealthy, overweight, obese body. The prevailing contemporary message communicated by the media and public health missives is that everyone everywhere is in the grip of an obesity epidemic. Calls to shape up and monitor one's weight and shape in an effort to avoid the life-threatening diseases avowedly caused by a few extra layers of fat are frequent. Those who already exhibit an 'overweight' physique are particularly targeted by these messages. However, as alluded to in the previous chapter, various body shapes and sizes have been considered desirable and undesirable throughout history. Perhaps the current obesity crisis is simply another fad with political, economic, and business agendas supporting it? Most health and medical professions would agree that human beings naturally fall into the bodily somatotypes of ectomorph ("skinny"), mesomorph ("muscular"), endomorph ("large") and their embodied bodily structures are not an indication of ill or good health. Consequently a number of health researchers throughout the world have questioned the contemporary preoccupation with obesity and the existence of an obesity epidemic. American academic Paul Campos states:

> *"The average American's weight gain can be explained by 10 extra calories a day, or the equivalent of a Big Mac once every 2 months. Exercise equivalents would be a few minutes per day. This is hardly the orgy of food binging and inactivity widely thought to be to blame for the supposed fat explosion. Whilst there has been a significant weight gain among the heaviest individuals the vast majority of people in the 'over-weight' and 'obese' categories are now at weight levels that are only slightly higher than those they or their predecessors were maintaining a generation ago. In other words we are seeing subtle shifts, rather than an alarming epidemic."*

So perhaps as a society we have simply been trained to focus on, single out, measure and scold those who don't meet the current socially constructed norm of the muscular-healthy body, more so than any other time in history. In such a context, obtaining a body that symbolizes good health and sexual desirability is often more important than having a body that is actually healthy. The main purpose of the grooming and body practices that these men have utilised is to achieve a body that is considered sexually desirable and healthy. This is a mission frequently reinforced by the mass media, popular culture and by private business, each of which seeks to profit from young men's aspirations and their body anxiety. Rocco and Jack discuss the various sources of information that have helped them to construct their knowledge in relation to the way they should look and the identities that they should present to their social worlds.

> "My partner. Friends...The guy environment and the media. I identified what I wanted to look like through the media. Magazines, advertisements etc." (Rocco)

*"[I] construct it based on the people I think are manly. Seeing other guys and trends, dressing like them and constructing my body physically like theirs. Don't read magazines so get it from real life. If I like the way someone looks or dressed I'll try imitate it...I know what I can and cannot pull off. I can't pull off all looks." (Jack).*

Both Jack and Rocco discussed the importance of the people that surrounded them within their social and cultural networks - at work, home, and in public. The bodies, appearances, identities and behaviour of their friends and of socially desirable strangers were considered good role models to observe and imitate. This process of self-reflection and self-surveillance in relation to others was critical to the process of constructing an identity that reflected contemporary social norms, trends and expectations. These young men sought and obtained an image, via various body sculpting practices that often showcased them as being masculine, muscular and sexually appealing to others.

Furthermore, Rocco surveills his body image through the glossy pages of men's fashion and health magazines. These magazines inform him of the latest fashion and fitness fads to ensure that his physique and appearance conform to the perceived social expectations that transfuse within his social nexus. He uses this knowledge to inform the bodily practices he engages in and he deliberately constructs specific personas, inspired by popular culture influences, using a variety of strategies and techniques to construct both the body and the identity he aspires to be and wants to present to the world. In effect, Jack and Rocco consciously manipulated the shape and appearance of their bodies to possess social, cultural, symbolic, physical and sexual capital to acquire and maintain the social criteria of an attractive healthy body and identity to establish levels of power and status within their community.

Although Jack and Rocco demonstrated some reflexivity, awareness and understanding of the various body and identity-changing practices they engaged in, and of what caused them to do so, Joe found it difficult to explain why he participated in the various body-altering routines. This lack of awareness is conceivably due to the affect of doxa, a learnt ignorance, and the dominant social messages that influence everyday activities (e.g. body maintenance and sculpting), which in essence help to construct perceived social realities and phenomena that appear self-evident and natural. These various messages are communicated and controlled by the media, the government, and by corporations and health professionals. They often influence the everyday citizen unconsciously by providing powerful social messages, expectations and pressure, often perceived as the truth, which may shape and govern the way that many young men appear and behave. In part, these hegemonic ideals may explain why many young men feel the need to construct the ideal masculine, healthy, attractive and muscular physique.

## Super Size Me

When young men are unable to attain a sexually appealing masculine 'aesthetic-athletic' body, many may start to look for alternative measures to reconstruct their lean or overweight bodies. These alternative methods can involve practices that enable individuals to obtain increases in muscle mass and perceived beauty, unachievable through traditional bodywork methods of weight training and high protein diets. The alternative body-altering strategy that surfaced strongly from this research was the use of anabolic steroids. Both Joe and Jack reveal in their personal stories how they and others used such drugs to create the body that they desired.

*"...main methods to construct [body] is gym and roids [laugh]...I don't take the roids these days to get bigger. I take it more to*

*maintain my muscle while I do cardio and help me to fine tune, which is why I don't take tren or deca [steroids]. [I use] Different drugs for different purposes. When I first started I wanted to get big and bigger. Over the last few years it's more about fine tuning and not wanting to go backwards [loose muscle]."* (Jack)

*"I consider it an investment....about twice a year...for 8 to 10 weeks. I originally wanted 85 [kgs]. Then it progressed too higher [120kgs] as my body composition started to change and I had to be more strategic and think long-term with my body. Well at the moment I'm carrying around a bit of fat...so when I lean down I will look beautiful. I'm allowing my body to grow stress free and being comfortable you know."* (Joe)

Both Jack and Joe deliberately used various types of steroids to manipulate the shapes of their bodies in order to acquire a form of physical capital that they considered desirable to themselves and others. Whether it be stacking on muscle or reducing surface body fat, their newly reconfigured larger, muscular and taught bodies were perceived to mirror characteristics of good health, fitness, strength, beauty and manliness: "I'm happier and healthier" (Rocco), "I used to be very fat and unhealthy so it definitely has a health benefit" and "It makes me feel healthy and improved my health" (Jack). Consequently, these outcomes and rewards, which were a direct result of the use of steroids, were seen as both short-term and long-term investments. For example, in a phenomenological sense, Joe perceives that using steroids has helped him to "Feel better about myself. Help me grow. To be the better me, for me." He regards his body as an unfinished product; an object that can be worked upon, modified and changed to create a body and identity that are better than they were both currently in the past. Joe feels that this experience and process can be attributed to the discourses of perfection modes and healthism that exist strongly within Western cultures. These various discourses reinforce the idea that in order to become something or someone, an individual must transform themselves from an "average Joe" into an identity that attracts attention, and stands out from the crowd in order to be seen and heard. However, the need to transform one's self often leads to many young men (and women) feeling insecure as their bodies do not measure up to the celebrities that they see on television, in glossy magazines, or in advertisements.

Negative psychological experiences were regularly raised throughout these young men's personal stories. Despite both men accumulating large amounts of muscle mass over a relatively short period of time - up to 40 kilograms of additional body weight - experiences of fear emerged at the possibility of losing the muscle mass that they had gained or/and at still perceiving that they were not muscular enough. Elements of paranoia and body addiction (body dysmorphia) had started to creep in, whereby they recognised that the physical, symbolic and cultural forms of capital that they had invested in could be lost or might remain un-achieved. As a result, these young men had arguably become addicted to various types of performance enhancing drugs (i.e. steroids) over the course of several years, in the pursuit of keeping up appearances.

The use of steroids to construct a physically desirable and self-gratifying body contradicted these young men's attempts to create a healthy body and to take care of themselves. Anecdotal and biomedical evidence would suggest that long-term and even short-term use of steroids can be detrimental to one's health and can also be potentially life threatening (e.g. various types of cancer; heart, liver and kidney failure), as the young YouTube sensation 'Zyzz', and many others like him have discovered. However, despite an abundance of anecdotal evidence from health professionals reporting an increase in the rate of enlarged hearts and kidney failure amongst seemingly healthy-looking young men, there is a lack of research to support these claims due to the various ethical implications of monitoring individuals who are on long-term (and short-term) doses of anabolic steroids. When I asked Jack and Joe if they had experienced any side affects from using steroids, they commented:

*"When using roids you feel...more edgy, short temper, but stronger and bigger, and that I'm achieving more." (Jack)*

*"When being lean all the time and taking all those chemicals [steroids] the stress it does to your heart and body and long term side effects...oh my god...but I've [gone] from lean machine at 59kgs too beefcake at 112 [kgs]...Well that Zyzz guy...always preaching "shredded" or you know gotta eat clean and lean... But he had a heart attack...I only [notice side affects] when I did a leaning out...made my heart jumpy and couldn't sleep... Steroids is often an emotional journey, when you come off...I live by the statement: If you can't handle your body off, you won't ever be able to handle it on, which means if you're not prepared to work hard when you're off gear [steroids] don't get on them at all. That's why a lot of people loose most if not all there gains [muscle]. They become reliant on the substance. Sure it helps, but not without hard work on and off the gear. But the things I've felt are. Bit depressed, emotional, insecure, but now I don't. I make sure I tell myself eat well train hard and you will be fine." (Joe)*

These insightful statements suggest that there are several physiological and psychological factors that are affecting their bodies and attitudes towards steroid use. Although these young men are aware of the potential pitfalls of steroids, and with the acknowledgment of the heart attack and death of Zyzz, and despite both personally experiencing increases in heart palpitations, an inability to sleep and a short temper, they still convince themselves that they can manage their bodies in a "healthy" fashion. Joe believes or attempts to believe that as long as he trains hard and eats well he will be fine.

One could argue that both these young men are deliberately ignoring the possible risks of using steroids, even when they have experienced symptoms of possible side affects, in order to ensure that they remain in a positive state of mind, enabling them to continue constructing masses of muscle. Joe's use of positive affirmations to influence his mind and behaviour, allowing him to effectively deny, ignore, avoid and reconstruct the truth or the perception of an event or experience, is a common human behaviour. Ty Hamilton, former teammate of Lance Armstrong in the Tour de France demonstrates this argument with his comment: " I lied for a long time...and you know – you start to believe some of your lies. I had been lying since my positive test back in 2004". And of course there was Lance Armstrong himself, who continually denied that he had ever used drugs or participated in blood doping, in order to ensure that he was still perceived as a champion in the eyes of the American public. Joe also has his thoughts on the reasons why many young men deny taking drugs for sports or/and beauty enhancement: "To me I think it's just a code. Denial, denial, but to some I think they want a bit of superiority. You know induce a thought of - yeah I did it without gear and they did. It's just a crock of shit". For Joe, Tyler, Lance and seemingly many other young men, the ability to believe their own self-talk and positive affirmations has become a coping strategy to block out information that they potentially perceive as detrimental to their bodies, identities, self-esteem and self-image. In Joe's mind steroids provide an opportunity to boost his physical and symbolic capital, as he can display the physical traits of macho-ness, strength, masculinity and beauty that have been achieved through hard work, dedication and superior levels of muscularity. Furthermore, Joe articulates how he overcomes feelings of depression and insecurity once he has completed a "cycle" of steroids:

*"When I first started I used to wear like four t-shirts as it made me feel bigger. Now I only wear one or two as some have holes in them...Not for body dysmorphia. I don't work out anymore for anyone else or for social gratification. If I did I would be leaner. Being big and beefy...yer don't cut it in the gay world, well in gay scene...pfffft anyway."*

To ease his experience of feeling anxious and insecure because he perceived his body to be too skinny, he adopts a coping strategy of layering his body with extra items of clothing to create a sense of a larger more muscular body. This is an emotional journey that he has accredited to his steroid use after he had completed a "cycle". His use of steroids seems to have perpetuated his struggles to accept and embrace the shape of his existing body. In spite of these heightened experiences he continues to construct his own reality, in regards to his perception of his body and identity. He continues to deny that he has "body dysmorphia" and justifies his body construction practices in terms of self-gratification, despite feelings of depression, he convinces himself of this mindset by stating that the "beefy" look is undesirable within the gay community.

Unlike Joe, Jack demonstrates some reflexivity regarding his social environment and makes the following observations about what influences his, and others' use of anabolic steroids in order to construct the ideal and socially desirable 'aesthetic-athletic' body:

> "...mostly to emulate the people they admire or find attractive or social setting like in Oz [Australia] it's a heavy rugby driven culture so you grow up playing rugby and need to be big but then the rugby boys look hot so you wanna look like them. Some do it for confidence and personal image. Some for sport, but a lot has to do with sexual attraction. Look at a firemans' calendar for example or rugby boys' calendar etc....you never find skinny people on there." (Jack)

Jack's testimony illuminates several social discourses, which appear to be significant in sculpting the minds and bodies of many young men. This statement provides an example of the cultural shift that has occurred in the last twenty years regarding steroid use. He suggests that the 'athletic-aesthetic' professional sporting body, which is often portrayed, idolised and glorified within the mass media, influences the way in which many male adolescents construct their bodies and also informs their individual body constructing practices. This shapes their perceptions of what a desirable, and consequently undesirable, body looks like. Traditionally, steroid use was restricted to professional athletes and bodybuilders seeking to out-perform their rivals, to receive large financial rewards, university scholarships and to advance their professional sporting careers. Their primary focus was not to look good. However, in the last twenty years, society has been increasingly exposed to the socially constructed attractive male sportsman's muscular and athletic body, which has been acquired by many male models, actors and entertainers. Progressively over the years these various bodies have become more and more revered and sexualised and they are now associated with attractiveness, sex appeal, desirability, romance, success and health. Therefore, a cultural shift has occurred: instead of increasing their sporting capital, young men now use steroids to increase their beauty capital. Jack states:

*"It is very commonplace for both party drugs and steroids. Sydney and other image driven cities, NYC, LA, London, the culture is very image conscious and very competitive…It's more competitive sexually speaking. It's also a summer city, has beach, sun, so there is a big emphasis on looking good with your shirt off."*

This statement would suggest that Jack feels the need to reconstruct and maintain what he, and many others within his social environment, perceives as a sexually attractive body which enables him to compete against other men in order to form relationships and to be accepted by others. This discourse of competitiveness is given as the primary reason for steroids within the community he interacts with. The use of steroids is seen as a way to acquire physical and sexual capital, a sexually attractive muscular body, which is perceived to increase his, and presumably others', power and status within social settings where men's bodies are often freely displayed.

The use of steroids by these young men to reconstruct their bodies has seemingly opened them up to various experiences of bodily pleasure and anguish as they seek to create the perfect body, to compete for the perfect partner and presumably to live the perfect life. So is it all really worth it?

## The (Dis) pleasures of a Disciplined Body

Historically, society has placed an emphasis on the de-pleasuring of physical activity. We hear statements like 'No pain, no gain' and 'Go hard or go home', which reinforce the idea that exercise and physical activity is hard work and not enjoyable. These discourses of displeasure were revealed within these young men's experiences of constructing a sexually desirable body, which included physical activity and various other bodywork practices. Jack and Rocco state:

*"...The maintenance and hard work and determination and limitation of foods etc. Need to be strict and disciplined - also it's expensive with protein, healthy food, gym membership and steroids" (Jack).*

*"I don't relax and enjoy life enough. I don't eat nice/fun food and I rarely party hard or drink...It should make you feel better than it does. Most people get so caught up in it that they don't even feel good when they look good and are too obsessed wanting and trying to look better." (Rocco)*

Within these two statements, discourses of the disciplined body emerge. These young men have deliberately sacrificed, restricted and limited some of the simple pleasures in life, like eating delicious sugary and fatty foods, socialising and drinking alcohol, so that they can reconstruct their bodies with controlled diets, regular weight training sessions and quiet nights at home. However, the disciplined body was not always perceived as a negative experience. Joe states:

*Creating and building...working...going to the gym...eating... its a commitment...sacrifice ...you have to appreciate what your body can do...not anyone else's...achieving and enjoying the goals your body brings......through hard work and determination......I eat six too eight meals a day...high protein and fibre and carbs...*

*sleep and train. There's nothing I don't like...I like everything, just growing, achieving etc.*

These contrasting perceptions and experiences of bodily discipline and control serve to illustrate the ways that individuals can create their own realities. Individuals can often perceive similar experiences very differently. While some enjoy the process of disciplining their bodies and can appreciate the physiological changes that occur, others perceive this experience as a necessary yet un-enjoyable process endured in order to get the body they desire. Clearly the feelings that they experience from this perception are unique to the individual. The young men interpret various situations differently depending on the world-views that they construct within their minds, which are often informed by their perceptions of the various social messages that filter through to them from their social surroundings. These in turn can influence the way they psychologically and physiologically enjoy or dislike their experiences at any given time.

Throughout history scholars have conceptualised the ways in which people and societies have manipulated their bodies using a diverse range of body-altering methods. These practices have been used to control, discipline, correct and improve the body for religious worship, battle preparation and war, improved health, the workforce, sports performance and of course for beauty. Sports historian Professor Douglas Booth states:

> *"...Holy asceticism increasingly became more fanatical and involved physical suffering... Christian asceticism gradually waned from the eighteenth century. But is asceticism really dead? Soldiers, athletes, dancers, weightlifters still over train and no pain no gain expresses their asceticism."*

However, prior to the early Christians, 2,000 - 2,500 years ago, the prominent Ancient Greek hedonists had a very different philosophy regarding the body. Booth states:

*"...The Greeks were hedonists and as such sought pleasure. The body was a key site of Greek hedonism with the Ancients holding relaxed attitudes towards sex and the consumption of food. The philosopher Epicurus (341-270 BC), for example, taught that pleasure is our first and kindred good."*

Despite having the ability to restrain themselves from the various temptations that surrounded these young men in order for them to discipline and shape up their bodies; much like the Christian Ascetics there was still a sense of un-fulfillment. Jack states:

*"...There's a constant feeling that it could always be better. In part it has for the sexual appeal and the ego, but where it hasn't to attract a sexual partner it's a feeling that maybe its not perfect yet...this is dependent on the feeling of the shallowness of the target audience. It definitely has boosted my confidence and I'm mostly content with it but always seek to improve it."*

Although Jack had made serious strides towards achieving the socially constructed ideal aesthetic, masculine and muscular body, he was still in search of what he perceived to be the ultimate, yet elusive pleasurable experience. The significant absence in his life was the pleasure of establishing and maintaining a sexual relationship with another person, which made him question whether the ideal body had been accomplished. Jack then contradicts himself, as he recognises the shallowness of this process, yet continues to participate in the various practices that enable him to construct a sexually attractive body. Perhaps the need to develop and maintain an intimate relationship with another is a product of our biological being and the physiological ability to procreate. Secondly, the need, want and desire to nurture a relationship with another person is reinforced within many cultures, to have a relationship, get married, have children and live happily ever after, barring the odd divorce. Consequently the perception of these young men to create a desirable, sexually attractive body in order to enter into a relationship is produced and reinforced through a multifaceted physiological, psychological and sociological process which leaves many young men doing whatever it takes to achieve the ideal romance that is glorified through popular culture.

In contrast to the various displeasures that these young men experienced, there were a number of perceived pleasurable experiences in working towards the ideal male physique. For example, all three young men suggested that modifying their bodies enabled them to acquire various forms of capital, resulting in increased attention which they enjoyed and which positively reinforced their decision to participate in numerous - and at times risky - body practices. For example, Rocco states: "I look better in clothes…and out of clothes… and I got to land a hot partner with an amazing physique." Joe and Jack also make similar comments: "It has boosted my confidence and I feel it definitely helps me attract the type of girls I'm interested in" (Jack) and "I love my ass, it gets a lot of attention, I like how people go nuts over it" (Joe). In these instances these young men reflected on how their well-sculpted and maintained bodies increased their physical, sexual and social capital. These young men perceived themselves to be more physically and sexually desirable due to the investments that they had made in their bodies. Their bodies had enabled them to acquire power and status within their socio-cultural spaces as they were now considered to be more attractive, and in Rocco's case this was suggested to be a key reason for the formation of his relationship.

Furthermore, Jack, Joe and Rocco experienced numerous other positive psychological emotions, which they attributed to constructing the 'aesthetic-athletic' body. Developing and maintaining increased amounts of muscle mass made them feel bigger, stronger, relaxed, happier, healthier and confident. Jack and Joe comment:

*"I feel big and strong by having more muscle and it makes me more confident. In a way it also gives a false sense of strength because even though you're bigger it's not necessary that you are functionally stronger." (Jack)*

*"Happy and confident...I like feeling strong." (Joe)*

Due to their reconfigured bodies these young men perceived and experienced themselves to be bigger and stronger, in both a physiological and psychological sense, which gave them more confidence within the social networks they interacted in. This feeling of confidence reflects the prestige that is associated with the male muscular body within their socio-cultural settings. These young men have attained symbolic capital through the size and appearance of their bodies and through their identity, which is seen to represent masculinity, strength, good health and attractiveness within the habitats they live. These positive sensations have been feasibly constructed socially through a multitude of sources that reinforce the described discourses. These young men's lives have been influenced by the dominant social messages that transcend through popular culture, including, health and educational establishments - particularly within the western world - that often portray the need for young men to behave and to appear strong, masculine, muscular and attractive. Consequently, when young men achieve these various manly characteristics it is no surprise that they embody a mindset and attitude that reflects a sense of achievement whereby confidence emerges from within them. Joe alluded to this sense of achievement, as he states: "I made it. It's mine. It's not for anyone else. It's for me. It's me. It's mine and if I choose to share it with someone or allow them in the process I will" and Jack: "It's a good way to de-stress and you feel healthy and you've accomplished something." These young men, had set out at an early age to deliberately reconstruct their bodies, influenced - consciously and subconsciously - by the various social messages that washed up, informing their knowledge of what it is to be an ideal man. In their eyes, and in the eyes of many glaring upon them, they have achieved their personal goals of attaining a body that is self-gratifying and socially admired. They can now proudly and confidently strut their stuff.

Interestingly enough the pleasures that these young men experienced having created the ideal male body and identity emphasised the various outcomes of working on and manipulating their physiques, as opposed to the process of their bodywork. Although they alluded to experiences of the 'phenomena' of pleasure during physical training, these pleasurable sensations were artificially created by various stimulants which included music and sports supplements. For example Joe states:

> "Yeh I use music I love my music...I use a pre-workout [stimulants] to give me that bit of energy that's about it...yeh it gives me a rush of energy...as I need to get it in when I've finished work and I'm dead it gives me the energy and drive to go to the gym."

This was a typical response from many young men, as not one person acknowledged any pleasurable sensations from simply exercising, dieting or from any other exercise or physical activity that they participated in. If anything, incidences of only anguish and sacrifice were discussed as they attempted to reshape and maintain their bodily appearance. The various body-constructing methods used were seen simply as a means to an end, which is of course, the aesthetic-muscular physique. Consequently this raises the question: Is it possible to experience pleasurable feelings of euphoria, adrenaline, pain, joy, vertigo, arousal and exhilaration when exercising and eating healthy food, or via any practice which is used to create a more appealing body and identity? What about 'runners' high', which has been described as an emotion of pure happiness and elation, a feeling of unity with one's self and/or nature, endless peacefulness, and a reduction in pain sensation following moderate and intense aerobic activity? These subjective emotions and experiences are similar to the claims of distorted perception, atypical thought patterns, diminished awareness of one's surroundings, and intensified introspective understanding of one's sense of identity and emotional status made by people who describe drug or trance states. And what about sensations of sight, taste, smell, touch, hearing, equilibrioception, kinesthesia and emotions associated with positive social relationships? The evidence provided by these young men would suggest that it is not possible to experience these pleasurable feelings through exercise, and indeed the scholarly research is not clear on this count. Many exercise scientists would argue that feelings of physiological pleasure are simply psychologically constructed and induced. That is, individuals perceive that exercise or healthy eating is beneficial to their well-being and body, which creates the perception of good health. Therefore, experiences of pleasure are psychosomatic. In other words, when a person perceives an experience (e.g. exercise) to be positive (or negative), then positive (or negative) thoughts are produced, which stimulate positive (or negative) neurochemical activity (i.e. release of endorphins) in the brain, which is in turn transmitted throughout the body. Put simply, you are what you think and you are the creator of your own personal experiences.

These young men experienced a range of psycho-physiological sensations, which were perceived and interpreted in various ways. The individual variations in these young men's experience of the various practices that helped shaped their bodies points to the importance of understanding how young men construct and make sense of the plethora of knowledge that informs their lives and their ways of being in the world. Ways of being that are socially constructed via the various social messages that filter through to them via their habitats, and ways of being that include their individual personalities, which may or may not be socially constructed. For example, the cynical, the optimistic, the introverted and the extroverted are examples of various personalities that conceivably affect the way in which a person perceives, interprets and makes sense of his/her own realities, truths, and his/her unique body and identity.

## Constructing the Individualistic Chameleon Body

The desire for these young men to construct an individualistic body and identity in order to reflect or/

and develop their individual personalities was a significant message that arose from their personal stories. For example, Joe states the reason why he places an emphasis on constructing a body that he perceives is unique to him:

> *Not fitting the mould...braving the storm...for what others think is not normal makes you more unique. It's not shown it's expressed....either through the way you dress, an opinion....the way you handle something...not conforming...The desire would be different for everyone. I just wanna be unique I guess not be like everyone else. So I guess the need to be an individual not be scared to create who I am.*

Discourses of individualism were drawn on by Joe in his emphasis on "being yourself" and in creating a body that allowed for "self discovery". Joe's need to find and express himself is feasibly influenced by popular cultural discourses that place an emphasis on bodies as unfinished projects, in need of constant work en route to perfection. These references can be seen throughout American popular culture, particularly with the rise of pop psychology and influential "life coaches" like Anthony Robins and Depak Chopra who attempt to help individuals to reach for the stars, to unleash and express their hidden talents from within and to strive for fulfilment by becoming all that they can be through various self-help books and seminars. Whilst many self-help gurus focus on the importance of focusing the mind in order to achieve success, corporations involved in fashion, television, entertainment, beauty and health focus on the body. Good-looking models, actors, celebrities and so called 'experts', supported by clever marketing and advertising campaigns, are used to promote and sell various products that make us look good, stand out. These products make us appear desirable - and of course unique - with one-off and limited-time-only products e.g. exercise equipment, jewellery, nutrition supplements, fashion items, cosmetics, beauty services, gym memberships and so on. However, as Anthony Robins and Depak Chopra will tell you, ultimately it's your ability to focus, believe in your natural talents and to act upon them, and not how good you look that will ensure that you achieve your goals.

Whilst Joe's testimony reflected a desire to reconstruct an individualistic body and to gain an identity that expressed his personality for perceived intrinsic purposes, Jack and Rocco's primary motivation for changing their physiques was to seek approval from others. Rocco states:

> "It definitely reflects my personality and the identity I like to create. It really is nothing like my natural body...Before [I reconstructed my body]...I couldn't get [other guys or girls] attention or pick up the guys that I wanted to."

Rocco has deliberately used a variety of techniques to reconstruct his body image, a body and identity that he now perceives as a more accurate representation of his personality. He likes to think that his refined body image suggests that he is an out-going, healthy, happy, successful and attractive person. Not only has Rocco created his body image through the shape and appearance of his physique, but also via his collation of various material goods, such as a sports car, nice clothes and a nice house. All of these reinforce his perspective of what makes a successful man. "A successful man should look physically in shape and have material positions that are inline with what he needs for his dreams." His need to create a body that portrays an image of wealth, success and personal achievement is socially fabricated through the hegemonic powers of private corporations and businesses that transmit the need for mass consumption and the purchase of their products, through various alluring attractive images in glossy magazines that evoke messages of happiness, fulfilment, opulence, health and beauty. Whether it be gym memberships, personal trainers, fitness magazines, skin care, fashion items or Ferraris, symbolism is used to attract and influence many young men in order to buy products that will help to construct a body and identity that is perceived to be desirable within the various social environments they operate. Rocco's newly fashioned image and identity has seemingly increased his physical and social capital, which has raised his social power and status within the community and enabled him to have more confidence in "picking up" another attractive and desirable mate, which he perceives has ultimately helped him to establish a relationship with his current good-looking partner.

Jack and Rocco both discussed how they used their acquired knowledge to sculpt their bodies, increasing their physical capital, which was attained through the various body altering practices that they participate in, in order to improve their careers. For example Jack states:

> *"I maintain a professional image...however I do leverage my physical appearance to my female customers...to my customers I need to be smart and tidy and dress well. I don't wear overly tight clothing...I might wear a slightly tighter shirt for a handful of my female customers that have a sneaky peak or seven! [laugh]... or maybe stand in a way that shows off more of my physique like cross arms [to give the perception of bigger arms and chest]. [I also] use it to draw attention to myself and satisfy my ego and definitely use it for sex appeal."*

Jack deliberately manipulates his body image to his own advantage. By revealing his muscular stature through tight clothing, unbuttoned shirts, and seductive postures to his female clients he uses sex appeal to help influence their decisions to buy his products. This sales strategy has the potential to increase his economic capital, power and status within the work force through increased sales. Consequently, he experiences his body in a positive way, with feelings of self-satisfaction and self-admiration, through the increased attention that he receives from the opposite sex.

Whilst Joe, Jack and Rocco suggested that their primary purpose for engaging in various bodywork strategies was to construct an

attractive and desirable appearance, the identities that they presented
to the world were not fixed. They would often experiment with
different identities, which showcased different personalities, moods,
feelings, beliefs and values. Joe demonstrates a degree of fluidity with
his identity as he provided various examples of how he transitioned
from one identity to another. He states:

> *"I think if I stay this immaculate person, all the time people
> would get bored of me. I like to look dishevelled and then be like
> BOOM when I go out. I like the idea of a transformation…
> evolution…my image had grown from bony boy with the emo
> hair…to pretty boy with the athletic physique…too blonde tanned
> god…hahaha ummm something I would have a wet dream
> about… but I wanted to look big bang theory crossed with jersey
> shore [television shows]."*

Joe's experience of fluidity and experimentation with his identity,
through the shape and appearance of his body supports the research
produced by developmental theorists who suggest that adolescence is a
period of time in one's life when a person searchers for their inner-self;
a time when they start to form their personal values, beliefs and
identity. Consequently, many young men seek out role models within
their social worlds to whom they can relate, observing and imitating
them in an attempt to create their own identity. From emos to sports
jocks, and from geeks to hipsters, adolescents often seek out singular
or multiple identities that they deem to represent who they are or who
they want to be. In an attempt to hide their changing, undesirable
and unbranded bodies, they create and try on individualised social
masks to see which ones fit the best. Joe is an introverted young
man, who prefers to spend time alone or with a select few as opposed
to spending his spare time in nightclubs surrounded by hundreds
of people. He describes himself as "socially awkward". However,
despite Joe's preference for quiet and peaceful spaces he deliberately
constructs a body and identity that enables him to express himself
physically, as opposed to verbally interacting with large numbers of

people, and draws upon popular culture celebrities and body builders for inspiration. In the following statement Joe continues to discuss the various influences that have provided him with inspiration to create an identity that allows him to freely express himself.

*"Kai Greene [body builder]...oh my god...for his determination and body. He motivates and inspires and I think he's an amazing human being...and I love Rhys Bobridge and Adam Lambert. Rhys - I just think he is the pillar of individuality and I find it alluring and inspiring I need to meet him. Adam – he's just amazing I love his look, similar to Rhys, but Rhys takes it that other level."*

These discourses and references from popular culture, such as entertainer Adam Lambert and body builder Kai Green, who have inspired Joe to construct an individualistic body and identity, arguably contrast with his unbranded body and identity. These performance identities appear to represent characteristics of extroversion with bodies that attract attention from others, which are often purely created for performance, sponsorship and business reasons so that celebrities and sports people can cash in on their talents. This is noticeable when you compare the young unbranded Adam Lambert that auditioned for 'American Idol' to the Adam Lambert that emerged afterwards, a young American talent that embodied a new era of glam-rock. This makes you question if these personalities really do reflect Joe's personality, identity and body and whether his attempt to construct an individualistic identity that represents who he is has really been achieved by his own accord. Or is he simply trying to make sense of himself through the body image of others instead of discovering who he is by utilising his own talents? Is this process of superimposing aspects of others' identities, predominantly drawn from popular culture really an act of individualism, or has Joe simply been seduced by capitalism and the commercialisation of numerous adolescent sub-cultures that are reinforced and consequently sold to the general public through the lenses of the mass media and Hollywood celebrities? Social researcher

Susan Cain suggests that we live in a world where the extrovert ideal has become the flagship of success, popularity and normality, which has consequently devalued the societal role and the benefits that introverts can contribute to the world as they are often perceived as weaker, less competent and abnormal. In reference to American culture Cain states: "We're told that to be great is to be bold, to be happy is to be sociable. We see ourselves as a nation of extroverts— which means that we've lost sight of who we really are". Consequently, introverts like Joe, who do not meet the desirable extrovert ideal are often made to feel inferior by their more extroverted peers and by the various mass media messages that promote extroversion throughout popular culture. The constant pressure to conform to the extroverted ideal often leaves many introverts exhausted, disheartened, and less effective in reaching their potential for success and in ultimately finding their true sense of individuality and uniqueness. As Joe begins to develop his reflexive abilities throughout the interview process, over a period of a few weeks he starts to use some of the skills associated with an introvert as he gradually begins to contemplate the origins of his desire to reconstruct his body image. He states:

> *"When I think about it more…prolly coz I never had that opportunity in high school to develop who I was because I was trying to stay alive. Suicide was always on my mind. I wanted to be strong on the inside and the outside. I can't be specific or tell you what induced that thought but that's something I can tell you now."*

Joe's harrowing school experience where he constantly felt harassed and isolated from his peers because of his introverted personality, his "skinny" frame and his "acne covered face" has had a significant effect on the way he perceives his own body. This experience influenced his decision to "develop" a stronger, muscular and masculine body. This desire to transform his body into an identity that was more socially acceptable suggests the need for him to hide and mask his skinny body and his introverted identity as an act of survival, safeguarding himself from the harassment of others within the social spaces he interacts with. To survive and overcome the judgement of others he deliberately set about acquiring physical and symbolic capital, by creating a body (and mind) that he perceived to be - and now experiences as - strong, with the ability to protect himself.

Although these young men experienced social pressure through constant surveillance of their various social worlds to live up to a socially constructed, accepted, desirable and ideal muscular-toned, acne-free and well-dressed body and identity, Rocco acknowledged individual variations on what was perceived to be an attractive and "fit body":

> *"There is more pressure in city environment. People are more image and material conscious than other smaller cities and towns, people care more about what they look like and, therefore, care more about what others look like. However, different 'scenes' require different looks. Not every scene requires perfectly fit bodies with perfectly manicured faces."*

As Rocco rightly points out, an individual's body image and his/her perception of what is attractive and desirable is subjective. Consequently, various "scenes" and social habitats require corresponding bodily shapes and sizes in order for an individual to be accepted within a particular community. For example, in contrast to the 'aesthetic-athletic' physique, there are numerous sub-cultures within both the heterosexual and gay communities. These include the "Big Handsome Man" (BMH), "Bears", "Chubbies" and "Foodees". British sociology scholar Lee Mohanaghan states:

> *"BHM…typically engage in processes of accepting and promoting their already sizeable bodies in a heterosexual space. A romantic or sexual focus is common…Bears engage in similar processes in gay male space. Although often considered more of an 'attitude' than a definable male type, Bears have a distinct symbolic style.*

*Their body schema incorporates full facial hair, an assured sense of masculinity and a level of body-mass typically equated with the ageing male body. Other types include gay male Chubbies. Typically more expansive than Bears, their expressions of self-acceptance are less assured. Others promote feeding and/or fattening processes, possibly with a sexual focus."*

Therefore, not all young men feel anxious about their existing large, overweight and hairy physical bodies, as they learn to embrace and become comfortable within their own skin. They learn to indulge in the pleasures of life, as they experience the rush of endorphins when they indulge in a delicious cream bun without the guilt of being perceived as a gluttonous, unhealthy, lazy slob. This is a pleasure that many young men are willing to sacrifice as they attempt to live up to social norms and expectations of embodying a healthy, fit and attractive male figure.

Whilst some men, like Joe deliberately experiment, refine and reshape their physical appearances to express their thoughts, beliefs and values and others simply embrace their bodies as they are, many young men not only conceal their socially flawed bodies, but also conceal their identities; in particular their sexuality.

## Alternative and Hidden Bodies and Identities

As Joe has grown older and experimented with his appearance, having escaped from the personally destructive confines of the school yard, he has used his body as an object of symbolic capital through which he expresses himself visually. He states:

*Well I always rock around in my gym shorts and high tops and a casual top...sometimes tsubi. I like that brand, as it has a casual emo appeal or I wear a pair of black framed glasses and slick*

*my hair back and look like a casual geek. I just like that they*
*give me an emo look. I see these creative little souls…that are*
*caught by societies judgemental view on them, and their only*
*escape, or expression is through their physical attire or face, hair.*
*I love it and think it's very brave as their look does not usually fit*
*mainstream. You know. And I think it's sad.*

In contrast to Rocco and Jack, who both seek to construct a desirable and normative body and identity that will merge in with their social environments, potentially allowing them to attain various forms of capital and to manipulate the various social habitats they live in by acquiring social power and status, Joe appears to do the complete opposite. Joe deliberately seeks to construct a unique and alternative appearance and identity that he feels symbolises the characteristics of mental and physical bravery, of strength and individuality, of creativity and of his journey to the overcoming of various negative life events. However, by acquiring an "emo" inspired identity that is often associated with being undesirable, abnormal and weird he potentially risks antagonising his social environment, which may result in further judgment, harassment and bullying from those that disapprove of his appearance within the social communities he interacts in. Therefore he is creating a social mask that could serve to alienate him from his social environment and potentially limit or even decrease his ability to acquire power and social status, in a similar way to his experiences as a "skinny" adolescent during his school days. This potential outcome appears to come to fruition when Joe comments:

*When I go to work I like to test them. I will stick a flower in the*
*side of my ear…they just stare at me and the staff are the most*
*discriminating, my kids don't even notice…some of the butchest*
*boys will ask me if they can wear it and I'm like sure but you*
*have to find me a new one and we have a laugh…but the staff*
*are like ughhh no wonder he gets bullied at work…or I get called*
*what I get called…cat cunt, poof, girl, shim, girl face, woman*
*body…I cop a lot.*

He deliberately tests the water within his working environment to
see the reaction he will get from his work colleagues as he experiments
with a variety of personas. Whilst some of the younger individuals
accept the alternative behaviours and appearances that he exhibits,
older conservative staff members discourage and criticise him as he is
perceived as being "gay" and "feminine". These perceived discourses
of feminine and gay behaviour demonstrate the social change in
acceptance towards homosexuality and the use of bodywork practices
that were previously perceived as female (e.g. wearing earrings)
within Western society. The younger generation appears to be more
open-minded about Joe's variance from the socially constructed
normative behaviours that a male should demonstrate in public,
whilst the older generation openly chastises his "abnormal" behaviour.

Whilst Joe seeks to test and express elements of his actual and
perceived personality, from his perspective many young men mask not
only their "abnormal" bodies, but also their undesirable sexuality. He
states:

> *"The ones that stand out are the two extremes...the overtly
> feminine and then there are the ones that are like awww yeah
> I'm straight-acting...and if you watch the straight-acting ones
> close enough you'll see them slip up and they turn into the
> biggest queens...and I love that...I don't judge em...and then
> if you watch the real camp [feminine] ones...watch em change a
> tyre on a car...its amazing...but I think out of both, the camp
> ones are being the most honest...Some are like what's socially
> acceptable...they would never let anyone see them singing show
> tunes or busting out to Christina Aguilera...they would die but
> I bet they have her blasting full ball in there ears."*

Arguably many young men are made to feel uncomfortable
within their own skin because of the socially constructed norms of
acceptable and expected male behaviour. These social expectations -
which are constantly present within young men's habitats - reinforce

the need for men to act masculine, strong and manly. Consequently, bodies and identities that are perceived to display characteristics of femininity and homosexuality are often condemned and stigmatised as being unnatural and unhealthy despite the apparent increases in social acceptance within western society towards individual difference. Therefore many young men consciously reconstruct themselves through various body and identity changing practices (weight training, fashion, diet etc) and unconsciously reconstruct themselves through social training whereby they observe and model themselves on the behaviours and practices of other males within their communities in order to exhibit masculine, heterosexual, macho, manly bodies and identities. These learnt and adopted ways are plausibly used as a defence mechanism to protect themselves from the judgment of others and to avoid being perceived as "queer", "sick", "abnormal", "risky" or "weird". Joe provides his perspective on the reasons why many young men create alternative "safe" identities.

> *"They'll be degraded if they're not...its a fear of not fitting in... and then once they do it so many times it turns onto autopilot... the camp ones are like fuck it...I've been fighting all my life... why let my guard down now...so they be themselves...the straight-acting ones are scared or they think they're better than the others. I think they are in this vision that they've survived the race to acceptance...its sad."*

Conceivably, as Joe suggests, many young men both consciously and subconsciously attempt to hide, recreate and self-regulate their behaviours, personas and identities in order to reflect and comply with the historical and socio-cultural norms within their social settings. As these young men are pressured by themselves and their communities into developing "normal" and "ideal" bodies and identities that restrict and mask their feminine, "gay", abnormal and deviant physiques, practices and identities, these adopted psyches often become autonomous and second nature. Consequently their socially perceived undesirable bodies, schemas, sexualities, personalities, and idiosyncrasies are sometimes only exposed to those people who they can trust and confide in.

The processes in which many young men engage in order to construct an ideal normative desirable body image are multifaceted and complex. However, despite individual differences, personalities, sexualities, body/identity practices and the various social influences that have informed their distinctive patterns of behaviour, their desires and objectives remain the same. Specifically, they have a need to attain an 'aesthetic-athletic' masculine body that is desired and accepted by all.

# CHAPTER FOUR

# Beauty and the Beast

Although many young men seem to explore, construct and experience different identities within their lives in order to obtain various forms of capital (e.g. social, economic and sexual), and also to manipulate and acquire power and status within various social spaces (e.g. home, work, social lives), as alluded to by Jack, Rocco and Joe, there appears to be one overriding identity that they aspire to embody....

## Act Like a Man!

The young men offered the following commentary in response to questions like: What does it mean to be a man? How should the ideal male look and behave? What makes a man desirable and successful?

Joe states:

> "...when I was growing up I was always faced with "this is how blokes do it", this is what men "should be doing"....I was always told if I did something wrong...It would be "you're a man act like it"....whether throwing a football, talking in a deep strong voice, making sure when I stand, that my hands were on my hips not my waist, as that would look too girly."

Joe, in the above commentary, reveals how the men who surrounded him during his childhood shaped his bodily behaviours, practices and identity. The way he performed tasks (e.g. sports, housework), talked, looked, and his posture, were all regularly observed, scrutinised, surveilled and modified to ensure that the characteristics of masculinity were represented. Any movements that were deemed "girly" and too feminine were quickly corrected and he was told to "act like a man". These taken-for-granted 'manly' behaviours and practices are often regarded as 'natural' and/or 'normal'. That is, many people perceive such practices of masculinity as being pre-determined by naturally existing physical and physiological characteristics - a person's genetics. However, Joe's testimony would suggest otherwise. Embedded in his comment is evidence that young men during their childhood reflect upon their so-called 'natural' body techniques; they can and do modify the techniques in relation to the social expectations of those in the socio-cultural environment within which they live. These social expectations or acts of masculinity are observed, taught, modelled, learnt and reinforced by other people that surround the young men. In other words, acts of masculinity are often socially constructed via the social expectations of others within the social spaces that people live.

American psychotherapist and social researcher Dr. Will Courtenay suggests that the aforementioned body techniques, geared toward creating a more masculine appearance, can become a compulsive practice, because they can be contested and undermined at any moment. This potentially means that the 'gendering' practices and behaviours of many young men become both habitual and defensive (often unconsciously) in order to protect themselves from being judged as less than masculine. Consequently, this process would appear to have affected many young men's perceptions of how men should behave and the body practices that they expect of themselves and others. This was evident in Jack's following statements:

*"...[men should] dress appropriately...like...they dress well and manly. Not a singlet down to their belly button or a handbag on their elbow groove...like when you look at them they look manly whether they're trendy or at the beach...in work gear etc.....or*

*they could be wearing a scarf but if they wear it right it looks good or they could wear it like a queen [in an overtly feminine way].*"

Jack is indicating the way that individuals are socially trained and gendered. He discusses how men should behave to ensure that their bodily appearance is constructed in a way that displays a masculine identity. He suggests that men should dress appropriately and be "manly" at all times; at work, at the beach and within other social environments. Discourses of heterosexuality and anti-feminine behaviour surface as he stresses the importance of dressing correctly in order to avoid judgment, and to avoid being perceived as a feminine "queen" as a result of presenting a non-masculine body image to the world he inhabits.

Furthermore, Jack points to the importance of embodying a cool, calm exterior to exude a masculine identity.

*"They [the ideal man] don't fly off the handle at little things... generally have a higher tolerance for things...not happy one day then a mess the other...have their head screwed on...they would be the person people would go to for support coz they're rational."*

Jack reinforces the need for men to behave rationally, and to keep their emotions under control. He stresses that it is important for men to be measured by their reactions to others and it is important for them to express themselves in an emotionally restrained and dignified manner. This need for young men to portray a rational body and mind - an identity that thinks and behaves in an orderly and logical fashion, is reflective of middle-class society discourses, which - as some sociologists argue - tend to mimic those of English society. The stoicism of the 'stiff upper lip', the resolute 'soldiering on' and the need to 'keep calm' in the presence of illness and suspicion are described as acceptable masculine traits by people who can trace their routes back to the United Kingdom as recently as a decade ago.

The avoidance of public (and even private) displays of emotion has been well documented throughout history. English historian Tony Walter suggests that the unwillingness of many men to discuss issues that expose their vulnerability, such as ill health, is highlighted in the most pervasive of human vulnerabilities – the inevitability of death. In the post-colonial, masculine culture, 'reserve and stoicism in matters of high emotion and the avoidance of undesirable subjects of conversation such as…death were normal.' Moreover, the demonstrative emotional expressions of grief were viewed as the business of women, not men. Sociologists McVittie and Willock suggest that this is because "men's understanding of health and illness are inextricably linked to other aspects of masculine identities, including the very notion of what it means to be a man", as alluded to by Jack. Scholarly research suggests that many men perceive their health and well-being as inseparable from their sense of their own masculinity. Perceptions of masculinity that embody and connect the solitary characteristics of mental, physical and emotional strength, and toughness to their health and well-being are expected to prevail. "That is to say that to be well is to be strong (i.e. masculine), and to be ill is to be weak (i.e. less than masculine)" (Rosenberg). This depiction of the manner in which many men, experience their own bodies and identities was hinted at during a presentation when a young man asked me if I would or had ever paid individuals to speak about their experiences of (re) constructing their bodies. His thinking was, 'why else would young men discuss their feelings and personal experiences, especially to a complete stranger?' To an extent he was right as numerous young men turned me down due to worries about being "psycho-analysed", presumably fearful of being prescribed as abnormal and, at one point, financial reward did cross my mind. The only reason I was able to gain the rich and detailed experiences of the young men that did take part in my research was because a level of trust and respect was nurtured.

Despite this strong sense of staunchness, these socially desired and reinforced practices of masculinity are often unique to the different socio-cultural and historical settings within which they occur and they depend on the acceptable masculine behaviour that prevails in any given location. "Notions of masculinity like notions of femininity are not static; rather, constructs of gender are constantly changing, with men and women not only subject to these changes but agents in effecting them" (Courtenay, 2000). For example French historian and scholar Morag Martin states:

> "By the late nineteenth century, physicians and anthropologists worried about the softening of the physical body in modern [French] society. The imperial project and the Franco-Prussian war were key moments in defining an unstable and highly criticized version of French masculinity. The French male was weak and overly intellectual and some even suggested that African colonials be recruited into the French army to reinvigorate it... French (elite) men have had 200 years of failing to live up to the iconic masculinities created by the Revolution and Napolean, while hanging on to the Old Regime vision of the civilized, intellectual gentleman."

This quote demonstrates that French masculinities were influenced over a period of time, within a specific social space (France) and by specific historical socio-cultural events and expectations that may have affected the way that many French men experience, construct and behave within their embodied selves. These French masculinities were possibly shaped by a changing cultural shift from the strong masculine military nous of Napoleon and similar political and military leaders during the early 1800's to modern and contemporary French masculinities which placed an emphasis on French men being seen to be civilized, intellectual gentleman.

## The Embodiment of a Nation

In contrast, societies outside of Europe like the Southern States in the USA and isolated countries like Australia and

New Zealand have witnessed the emergence of a consistent dominant type of masculinity. These masculinities seem to place an emphasis on men's embodiment of strength, toughness, authority, leadership and 'manliness' which can be seen in the way that they express and experience their bodies, minds and identities. These characteristics clearly surface in the three young men's testimonies as they discuss what it means to be a man and how an ideal man should look and behave:

> "...powerful, strong and the provider in a relationship. He should look muscular and masculine...A man should be confident, strong, powerful and brave. A man should be the protector and provider. A man should inspire and lead." (Rocco).

> "...be strong and confident, have testicles, not wear a dress... reasonably emotionally stable...be confident and control of situations where a decision needs to be made...take responsibility for their actions..." (Jack).

These young men's desire to perceive the ideal man as one that embodies the physical characteristics of strength, power, muscular, bravery and masculinity transcended their individual differences in social class, cultures and ethnicities. These characteristics are represented throughout history and have formed the core of an "acceptable" man's credentials, which have been passed down through the generations and through various male role models. During the early 1900's nationalist discourses produced the citizen soldier as the exemplary citizen, in many American states these discourses still reign true. Throughout the world the soldier provided the perfect role model for young men as he symbolised courage, bravery, strength, toughness, self-sacrifice and resolve as he represented and fought for the freedom of his country. The prestige ascribed to soldiers was derived from their alleged procreative role as a result of their courage and bravery at Gallipoli on 25 April 1915. Australian historian Marilyn Lake discusses the importance of the Gallipoli war and how it helped to define a nation and its citizens:

> *"Australia had had her birth and her baptism in the blood of her sons'. They had displayed manly qualities, 'a feat of arms unparalleled in history'. Indeed it quickly became evident that the Anzacs were not merely manly, they approximated to the status of supermen. They showed a spirit of manly qualities, said General Birdwood, 'that had never been surpassed in the annals of arms'. 'Gallipoli would stand as a symbol of great deeds greatly wrought, a place where the courage, strength and endurance of our southern manhood was put to a supreme test and did not fail.' At Gallipoli, Australia 'had leapt from the cradle of her nationhood into the front rank of the bravest of the brave."*

These discourses of nationalism, war and heroic masculinity still play an important role in Australian and American culture today. From the social expectations of older generations who have conceivably reinforced these militant character traits (subconsciously and/or consciously) in their children, (the young men of today), to the large public monuments dedicated to the war dead and veterans that dominate cities, along with the thousands of small memorials that mark the landscape. Symbolisms of nationalism and masculinity are celebrated with the commemoration of National Holidays, whereby men and women, young and old, remember and salute their heroes of yesteryear. Consequently war heroics and heroes have seemingly played an important role in shaping the identities of many young men throughout the world. The enduring hegemonic masculine discourses, of strength, courage, bravery and leadership have plausibly provided a social blueprint for many young men and provided them with an identity to look up and aspire to.

This sense of nationalism and national pride that many young men embody, through symbolic capital, was evident during my three years of teaching in Australia. I observed that many young men - mostly from working class families - either possessed or desired tattoos. The tattoos that numerous young men had or wanted represented the stars on the Australian national flag, the Southern Cross. This phenomenon can be witnessed up an down the sun-drenched beaches of the Australian coast line, during Australia Day (January 26) and during one-day cricket matches where young Australians showcase their national pride through their tattoos and bodies, often accompanied with the chant – "Aussie Aussie Aussie, Oi Oi Oi." However, for many Australian youths this act of symbolism represented more than being a proud Australian. Rather, it represented elements of racism, anti-immigration and the support of a white Australia. I was often dismayed at the racism within my classroom, as many young men (and women) would demonstrate feelings of hatred towards non-white Australians. On my second day of teaching, students boasted of white Australian supremacy as they showed me video clips of the Cronulla riots. The riots were an infamous moment of youth racism in Australia's history where large groups of young white male Australians aggressively attacked people of color. So how did these feelings of hatred emerge towards non-Anglo-Saxon Australians? To put these discourses of nationalism and anti-immigration into context, Lake offers some historical insight into this issue:

> *"As immigrants…British Australians were anxious about the future of their race and their ability to hold the continent. The long coastline and 'vast empty spaces' heightened the young nation's sense of vulnerability. Their proximity to the numerous peoples of Asia simply accentuated feelings of isolation and the insecurity of this outpost of Empire…As colonizers and colonized both, Australians of British descent committed themselves to the establishment of a White Australia. This necessitated a denial of the existence of Aboriginal Australians who were cast in the role of a 'dying race' and severe restrictions on the entry into Australia of non-white foreigners…[which] prevented undesired immigrants from settling in Australia."*

These historical fears of immigration and the need for white Australians to assert their control over non-English immigrants – in particular 'Wogs' (Mediterranean immigrants), Asians and Muslims seems to have continued into contemporary Australian society. An Australian blogger provides us with his perspective on young Australians and racism:

> *"The rise in xenophobia, racism and rampant jingoism in this country can initially be traced back to pandering to redneck independent MP Pauline Hanson and her brain-dead supporters back in the mid-90s. Add to that the growing ill-will towards Muslims after 9/11, followed by the Tampa/children overboard scandal in 2001 and you could see where things were heading. Then came the Cronulla riots in December 2005, a shameful day in this nation's history. Idiots running amok, attacking non-Anglos on the beach, in trains. It was a fucking disgrace. It wasn't a coincidence that a few weeks later – on Australia Day 2006 – came the first news reports of groups of Anglo teenagers wearing Aussie flags round their neck (the so-called "Cronulla cape") forcing non-Anglos to kiss the flag while proudly displaying inane slogans – "You flew here, I grew here!", "Fuck off, we're full!" – scribbled on their bodies with zinc cream."*

Evidence of this can be seen in the political and social tensions that have been created recently with the arrival of 'boat people' who have sought asylum in Australia from Sri Lanka since 2011. An English journalist states "The impact on the Australian psyche has been significant, with half of the public seeing the issue as more or equally important as issues of managing the economy, education and health services". This unhealthy anxiety towards immigrants - past and present - appears to be affecting the way that many young people in Australia express themselves and it has had a significant impact on the presentation of their bodies and on their individual subjectivities.

## Tall, Strong, Sportsman

Strong discourses of hegemonic masculinity and nationalism continued to emerge in other forms within Joe's, Jack's and Rocco's social spaces through the analysis of the young men's personal stories. Images of powerful, strong, muscular, confident, leaders in sport surfaced, which appear to have shaped their preservation of the ideal male, and consequently the way that their own bodies and identities should look and behave. Joe makes the following comment when he reflects on what he considers to be the ideal male persona:

> *"To be strong...To be masculine...to be protector. [Like] Tall, strong, sportsmen. Big shoulders...strong arms...look like they carry the world on there back...Rough."*

These discourses of masculinity and their association with the sporting body provide an insight into the Australian psyche, and the value that is placed upon the masculine-athletic body - a desirable schema that Joe and many other young Australian men are influenced by. Australia is a proud sports-playing nation and sport has played a crucial role in defining their culture and way of life. From rugby to cricket, from Australian football to a long history of Olympic legends, sport runs through the veins of many young Australian men and plays a significant role in defining their identity both as a nation and as individuals. Over the years international sporting performances and events have provided Australians with a source of immense national pride as they have competed, excelled and often dominated more economically and politically powerful nations on the world stage. Thus, sport has given Australia a sense of identity and the ability to showcase its athletic abilities, its sporting prowess its stadiums, technology, culture and its land of golden soil which abounds in nature's gifts, beauty rich and rare to the world. Thus, numerous young Australian men hold the sporting anatomy in a positive light and the athletic-sporting body is often highly sought after.

The desirability and attractiveness of the strong, muscular sporting body is socially constructed through the Australian media. Sport, by and large, is still free-to-air for most Australian households, and the muscular athletic male physiques of rugby league and Australian rules football players dominate prime time television during most afternoons and evenings, Friday to Monday, and during the occasional mid-week blockbuster. Weekly news media reports quickly follow, along with any news stories or scandals about the nation's favorite masculine, muscular and attractive sporting heroes. Successful Australian sportsmen are held up as national icons. Bradman, Thorpe, Lewis, Laver and Eales have all received national accolades and capital in the form of statues, stadiums, awards, financial wealth, and social status in recognition of their athleticism and leadership. It is hard to live in Australia and not notice the tall, strong, typical sportsman that surrounds you via the media or in person. This figure is one that shapes many young men's perceptions of a desirable body. What young man would not want to be perceived as attractive, famous and successful with a beautiful young 'WAG' (sportsman's Wife And/or Girlfriend) on his arm?

Historically, sport in Australia - and indeed many other nations throughout the world - has been used to groom and develop young men to become more masculine. Many club and school sports, and physical education lessons, were created to achieve the objectives of instilling the characteristics of toughness, fitness, discipline, competitiveness, leadership, confidence, communication skills, teamwork and mate-ship within young men. Increased experiences of feeling more masculine as a result of playing sport were revealed when Joe and Jack discussed playing rugby. Jack stated:

> *"....playing rugby [union] made me feel stronger and [I felt] empowered being able to play a highly physical sport."*

Furthermore, Joe shared his recent experiences of his first club rugby league game:

*"My body is destroyed. From the rugby [league] game. I'm sore all over and I feel more masculine. Not even lying. First half no one would run at me. I was on the wing...my team mates said, "they don't know you, you haven't played before"..."They think you're too big." Then I finally got hold of the ball and leveled three of [th]em and made some ground. And I got creamed a few times. It was a good experience...[I felt] strong like bring it on mother-fuckers...being able to physically justify it on queue was great...[I felt more masculine] Coz I thought they were going to be homophobic or pricks..... But I couldn't pick up on anything...I was just playing the game...I made it VERY clear I was gay. [I] just felt more accepted, like yeh I'm gay but ummm they def judged me as a man first."*

Both these young men discuss their positive experiences of playing a contact sport and the effects it had on their bodies and identities. They experienced heightened feelings of joy, empowerment and pleasure in using their bodies to compete against others physically. Interacting physically, tackling, smashing and colliding with others produced feelings of increased masculinity. They felt stronger and gained satisfaction from unleashing and successfully executing acts of aggression towards others in a controlled manner. Were these young men's experiences of bodily pleasure and satisfaction in producing aggressive acts of behaviour induced through participating in acts of physical body combat? Or was it a natural outlet for these young men to set themselves free from the socially constructed, well-mannered, norms of behaviour? Many psychology and psychiatry scholars would argue the latter; that many young men are naturally more aggressive. American psychiatrist Robert Burton states "Masculinity is operationalized primarily by the male hormone, testosterone. The presence of this hormone circulating in the blood stream has a large influence on the degree of aggressive behavior that an individual will exhibit". Therefore, one could argue that sport and exercise provides a controlled environment in which young men can learn to manage their anger and aggression in a healthy fashion. In any sport, effective use of a player's aggression is easily identifiable, whether it exists in the form of a 'home-run' or a tackle. On the other hand, overly aggressive behaviour is normally not allowed, and is penalised. Furthermore, Burton states:

> *"Through sport, an individual athlete's psychological development can be promoted and perpetuated. As child, adolescent, and adult development continue, an optimal zone around sport and its attendant aggression should facilitate and further the capacity to be appropriately aggressive in life's many challenging situations. The experiences of sport should then lead people to be able to generalize their experience to other social contexts, in which it will be beneficial to either express or restrain their aggression. Guided and assisted by attentive parents, coaches, and significant others, involvement in sport offers promise for all kinds of athletes, in contrast to current impressions of arrested development and pathology among athletes. Viewing aggression in its healthy form, in contrast to its extreme and inappropriate versions, and sport as a health-promoting exercise in psychological development and maturation may allow participants and spectators alike to retain an interest in it and derive further enjoyment from it."*

This notion that many men have a biological predisposition to aggressive behaviour, more so than females, reinforces the socially constructed gender stereotypes. These gender discourses suggest that men are masculine, strong and tough and females are feminine, gentle and weak. However, we have all seen these stereotypes dismantled in everyday life as female Olympic champions and gold medalists exhibit characteristics of strength and power, whilst many men demonstrate ostensibly female qualities such as beauty, slimness, sensitivity, speaking softly, physical weakness and emotional displays.

These are feminine characteristics that Joe once embodied. However, through engagement in various body constructing techniques, he managed to reconstruct his body into an image of masculinity - a body that reflected the characteristics of strength, power and toughness through acquiring increased muscle mass. This process, consciously or unconsciously, provided him with the physical and symbolic capital he now embodied, as he had a physique that was accepted by other masculine and muscular men, which led to him being invited to play a game of rugby league. Joe stated, "they asked me [to play rugby league] due to my size and speed at work". However, Joe's newly created stronger, powerful and muscular body did not prevent him from experiencing feelings of apprehension and anxiety about playing since he anticipated possible feelings of rejection for his sexuality. The other players eased his anxiety after his first game of rugby league as he felt that he was treated equally and accepted by the other players. Joe's reconstructed masculine and muscular body had enabled him to overcome gay stereotypes by acquiring physical, symbolic and social capital. He had become accepted by acquiring power and status within this particular social network by securing a body and identity that reflected the characteristics of the ideal masculine man. This was a far cry from the skinny acne-covered adolescent that once felt harassed, bitter, resentful, and unaccepted by his peers.

The respective sports that Joe and Jack participated in also afford a sense of the way in which their individual bodies, subjectivities, practices, and knowledge are constructed within the social 'worlds' that they live. Evidence of Jack's middle-class background is represented by his participation in rugby union. Australian and British education scholars Richard Light and David Kirk comment:

*"Elite independent schools are typically characterized by the preservation of tradition and explicit efforts to connect to current practice with a past that confirms as institutions serving the privileged. There has been a historical emphasis placed on sport as a means of distinguishing GPS (Private Schools) from government schools since their inception that has seen them operate as masculinizing institutions for the ruling class.*

*Within this context rugby has long operated as both a practice of distinction and as a means of inculcating a particular, class specific for of masculinity connected to Victorian/Edwardian ideals of 'manliness'.*

These ideals of manliness are based upon a firm belief in the moral dimension of sporting activity, particularly through an involvement in rowing and rugby. "Their primary purpose was 'to create a universal Tom Brown: loyal, brave, truthful, a gentleman and, if possible, a Christian" (Mangan). The discourses of a middle class masculinity, which are embedded within private schools, seemingly play an influential role in shaping individual identities and the bodily practices they engage in. Thus, the ideal middle-class social body and identity is taught to exude and symbolise elitism, success and gentlemanly behaviour.

In contrast, Joe's participation in rugby league speaks to his working class background. Rugby league was established as a sport for the Northern English working class in 1895, followed by Australia in 1907, as a result of a schism between the upper class, who controlled the sport of rugby (union), and the working class, who could not afford to take time off work to participate in rugby. Consequently, the working class established their respective rugby leagues. English sociologist Richard Hoggart discusses how working class men achieved a sense of 'symbolic citizenship' and a sense of pride through their allegiance and association with local teams in his successful novel 'The Good Companions'.

*"Ruby league in the local area became the leisure time focal point of a masculinesed 'us', a demarcation point not only from the drudgery of work hours, but also the 'authoritarianism' of the general 'public life' associated with 'them', the bosses and their cohorts in civic officialdom."*

Furthermore Hoggart suggests that the construction of the 'masculinised us' identity was for the working class and further exaggerated with the association of masculinity and alcohol.

*"In the north of England the local ales were presumed stronger and became a status marker of tough masculinity against a comparatively inferior and insipid beer from the southern counties. This simplistic binary view of strength and weakness extended to football and even cricket as northerners believed their teams to be tougher and therefore in possession of the greater competitive spirit. The emergent symbiosis between supporting sport and consuming alcohol further entrenched the masculinity of sporting culture."*

These masculine practices and rituals are firmly entrenched within English and Anglo-saxon working class cultures. For many men, constructing the rough and tough masculinities of the working class is strongly visible as they play or/and watch with their neighbours, friends and workmates in fields, stadiums, sports clubs, bars and homes up and down the country, accompanied with a few (or many) pints of beer. In effect, their masculinity is affirmed as they demonstrate who is stronger and tougher with big 'hits' (tackles) and big drinking. Although Joe may not have fully participated in these masculine sporting practices, growing up in a society where these discourses are privileged has plausibly shaped his knowledge and perceptions of an ideal man's appearance and how he behaves.

The socially constructed masculine, sporting and drinking life is an important part of the culture that Joe was embedded within. It perspires through many, if not most, young working class males' bodily pores. Consciously or unconsciously, it seems to shape their perceptions of what is considered to be the ideal male identity and body. One's class and interactive social spaces often influence these masculine sporting schemas and bodies. Obtaining the perfect match of the desirable and acceptable body within one's social environment is crucial in acquiring power, status and capital (social, cultural and physical) as illustrated by young Joe's sporting experience.

## From Scary and Monstrous to the Pretty 'Aesthetic-Athletic' Body

Despite the dominance of the historical discourses of the strong, tough, masculine sporting male, particularly within the rugby, wrestling and American Football youth and adult male cultures that dominate in many masculine driven cultures throughout the world, there is seemingly a shift at work in how many young men construct their bodies and identities. This shifting sense of what constitutes a desirable body image could conceivably be attributed to a change in the social messages concerning health, wealth, fame, popularity and beauty within these young men's individual social environments.

In a discussion with a young man, Troy (28), who lives in a working class neighborhood and manages a sports nutrition shop in an affluent area closer to the city, I asked about his perceptions of young men's body image. He stated:

> "[In] my opinion... the gap is being breached. There was probably an obvious difference years ago but now the lifestyle/body wanted is the lean-aesthetic type. West boys: bulky, strong all about max weights lifted...on average...rougher upbringings / gangs / stigma was the bigger the better the scarier taut and masculine...more of a statement. East boys: surfy, lean, fit, cardio was emphasized. Now the west and east has merged to the middle of both."

This young man's perception of the environments he lives and works in provides an insight into the body that he perceives many young men desire and into the changes that have occurred within and across social classes over recent times. This comment highlights how young men in the working class suburbs use the body-constructing practices of weight training, tattoos, growing facial hair and the avoidance of grooming to create a body and identity that symbolises the characteristics of fear, toughness and masculinity in order to make a statement which will intimidate others and ward off any potential threats, thus protecting themselves, their loved ones and their territories. The need for men to create these scary and masculine bodies and identities was attributed to the social spaces they lived in. The living environments of the often-neglected working class areas were perceived to increase many young men's chances of being exposed to violent and potentially life-threatening situations, as young men grew up surrounded by gangs and family abuse, in addition to poor housing and living conditions. From my personal experience of teaching in the rough working class inner city schools of London, I noticed that it was not only the hardened, street-wise students who tried to display the behaviours of male bravado, but also many young male teachers. Young teachers would often grow facial hair and beards to make themselves look older and more masculine, ostensibly to control who they perceived to be potentially unruly students and to prevail in the wars of the classroom. Young male teachers sought to construct a body image that reinforced and established control, dominance, toughness, no-nonsense, wisdom, seniority, and respect.

In contrast to the rough, tough and scary bodies of many working class suburbs, the bodies of those in more affluent suburbs were perceived by Troy to be fit, lean and healthy. The suburbs in the East of Sydney, where I taught for several years, have been traditionally associated with Anglo-Saxon middle class professionals, where the houses are located in prime locations, which provide easy access to the sand, surf and sun. Differences in body image based on class and geographical location were reinforced with Jack's statement:

*"[The ideal man] stays active and keeps fit…Physically healthy…*
*Think its symbiotic with being energetic and mentally healthy.*

*[He has] energy, drive...passion, intelligence, ingenuity. They*
*have a goals and are passionate about it...Energetic not lazy and*
*sit on a couch day dreaming...They make things happen."*

Jack's comment suggests a multitude of discourses that influence
his and other young males' middle class bodies, identities and
masculinities. These discourses allude to the various social messages
that surround young men via popular culture and to the relationship
between a healthy and fit body and personal success. On this basis,
the ideal and successful man embodies the personal traits of passion,
intelligence and the drive to succeed, which is performed and attained
via a physically and mentally healthy body. Prominent sociologist
Raewyn Connell argues that this urban middle class masculinity is
a version of masculinity organised around dominance, emphasising
"leadership" in management and/or expertise, and also emphasising
"professionalism" and technical knowledge. The symbolic capital
acquired through presenting a "professional" and healthy attitude,
body and identity to the social milieu, which young middle class
men interact with may lead to prospective employment and career
opportunities. These opportunities may increase one's ability to
acquire power and status in addition to economic and social capital
within their profession and possibly within wider social circles. This
is a process and achievement that many young professionals value en
route to obtaining an image that represents the "ideal", healthy and
successful man.

Continuing on from Troy's previous statement, he suggests that
these middle class discourses often portrayed by young men in the
traditionally affluent suburbs have started to have an influence on the
bodies of young men in the West. Furthermore, Troy, states:

*"The west working class image has shifted. These days there are*
*top of the line schools in west, good jobs etc. These days kids/guys*
*etc. want to look good, and shredded [toned] to go out, feel good,*
*pick up girls etc. The image of bulky/big is out so the trend now is*

*to look a certain way and doesn't matter where you are everyone
tries to follow that trend. It's about the pretty factor these days...
he [Zyzz] was a big influence on today's kids to look normal, lean
and muscley rather than monstrous."*

His personal experiences and observations provide an insight
into the social change that has influenced the way in which a number
of young men currently experience their bodies and identities. In
his mind there has been a clear shift from young men wanting to
obtain large intimidating scary bodies in order to protect themselves,
to a muscular 'aesthetic-athletic' body which makes them look good,
feel good and be desirable to the opposite sex. He perceives that this
cultural shift has been influenced by the physical and social changes
that have occurred in the various suburbs of the West over recent
times. The development of private schools, a university, apartment
buildings, increased businesses and leisure facilities, combined with
improved transportation systems to and from the city, all seem to
have had a positive affect on the area and the people that live there. It
would appear that certain areas within the western suburbs are now
safer places to live, with increased prosperity and the opportunity for
individuals to overcome the associated problems with poverty (e.g.
increased gangs and violence, criminal activity, poor housing and living
conditions, and poor health). The re-development of these working
class communities, through public and private investment, has seen
a change in how many young men in the west see, experience and
present themselves to the world. While many young men, particularly
within working class neighborhoods, still demonstrate the traditional
tough, rough masculine bodies and identities, other young men in
the West have begun to use various body practices to create a new
type of working class masculinity. These young men have started to
reconstruct an 'aesthetic-athletic' masculinity by consuming healthier
foods and sports nutrition products, by accessing fitness centers, and
by paying greater attention to men's fashion and grooming products
and services. All of these activities were previously seen as too "gay" for
the butch, tough, scary men of the west and were thus limited to the

middle class white guys in the eastern suburbs. Therefore, the number of young men in the west who currently use their bodies socially, culturally, economically, symbolically and sexually has significantly changed in contemporary times.

Whilst Troy perceives that there is less of a difference in the way that young working class and middle class men construct and present their bodies to the world, when comparing the current generation to those gone by, the knowledge, influences and experiences that inform their individual identities and their appearance are often significantly different. As discussed previously the social environments that people live in, which themselves are often influenced by the prevailing social class, can play an important role in shaping an individual's identity, physical appearance and lifestyle. These individual differences have been presented in each of the three young men's personal stories. From the violent, abusive and rough working class environments in which young Joe was brought up to the middle class experiences and expectations of success, intelligence and professionalism that shaped Jack and Rocco's behaviour, body image and individual masculinity.

However, although these young men, and many others, display personal behaviour and masculine identities that are arguably influenced by the various social messages within their social spaces via their social class during their upbringing, the 'aesthetic-athletic' muscular toned body that they seek to embody would appear to transcend these individual cultural and class differences. Jack, Rocco, Joe's and Troy's testimonies, and the insights and experiences of myself and others that I have alluded to, would suggest that there are universal influences and social messages displayed by young men throughout today's world that affect their body, identity and masculinity construction. Individual's bodies and identities exist within a complex system of socio-historical influences, expectations and discourses. The media, along with culture, class, politics, health and gender, all affect many young people's behaviour; their sense of identity and of their appearance to others. However, individual bodies and identities are not merely socially constructed by the multitude of the various expectations and the perceived natural ways of acting like a man that inform their unique personal practices and behaviours. Individual identities are also influenced by their physiological states of being; their sex, sexuality, sexual desire, age and personalities are all factors which may influence their perception of these socially constructed norms of behaviour. On the one hand, a person's perceived 'natural' body and identity may be unconsciously suppressed in the face of the social messages that surround them; on the other hand, some people rail against these messages, letting their existing and sometimes hidden behaviours, bodies and identities show, even when they risk being considered abnormal, weird or different due to their non-conforming bodies, identities, practices and behaviours.

# CHAPTER FIVE

# From Obsession to Acceptance

## Key Insights

These young men's personal stories and insights provide us with an understanding of how young men perceive, construct and experience their bodies in contemporary society. They afford insights into the plethora of influences, events, motivations and emotions that affect young men's perceptions, and the development and presentation of their bodies and identities. They point to the varied ways in which many young men take up and internalise (or not) 'body' knowledge that is circulating in their specific social contexts and the way in which they use various body techniques to attain a socially desirable body. They also air the rogue, resistant attempts of some young men in the face of the ubiquity of ideal body messages. For example, Joe's struggle against social norms and expectations to create what he perceives to be an individualistic body that expresses non-conformity. However, their familiarity with dominant discourses concerning masculinity and what qualifies as an 'ideal' body inevitably influenced and constrained the way they portrayed themselves within various public spaces (e.g. work, school, home, nightclubs). Consequently, each of the young men, like millions of other young men around the world, engaged in some form of bodywork with a view to attaining a specific kind of body, and consequently attaining an identity that is considered attractive, healthy, manly and ideal within the social settings and spaces they live.

Yet, as their stories suggest, adolescent identities are complex and multi-dimensional, constantly undergoing a process of constant negotiation and renegotiation. Their perceptions of important matters, their understandings of whom and what they are and what they might become morph over time, and upon reflection. Jack and Rocco demonstrated that an awareness of "social body trends" - which were used to mask their biologically undesirable bodies - was beneficial to their lives, their careers and beneficial for building relationships with others. These young men negotiated their way through their social worlds by acquiring a desirable appearance and identity that enabled them to manipulate their social networks by acquiring power and status as a result of shaping up to social expectations of the ideal man. In return, these young men were often rewarded with social, cultural, economic and sexual capital, for example increased public attention, improved sales and sexual relationships. However, wearing a superficially imposed body and identity, and living up to social ideals often comes at a cost as it shields our natural idiosyncrasies and personalities from those whom we do not know or trust in order to protect ourselves from judgment and rejection. This limits our ability to connect meaningfully and to bond with others. These alternative identities not only mask our naturally "risky" selves, they sometimes totally consume the way that some young men perceive themselves, ultimately losing touch with the person they once were. Their alternative bodies and identities become habitual, second nature and permanently embodied. In other words young men, and women, learn to judge people by their covers and in the process often become and define themselves by their own external facades, which they have constructed. Consequently, many young men like Joe, Jack and Rocco become entrapped by the superficial body that they have constructed and yet feel that they need to retain. The fear of rejection on the grounds of being too fat or too unattractive is an emotion experienced by many young men and women, it is a fear that feeds their self-conscious minds and keeps them motivated to keep up with their appearances in order to ensure that they embody a physique that is both socially desirable and acceptable.

Alternatively those men like Joe who struggled with their identities, frequently seeking to challenge pre-existing bodily and identity norms by constructing alternative identities (e.g. an emo), or those who maintained their "skinny" or "fat" bodies were often perceived as unhealthy, unattractive and undesirable, and they were frequently subjected to social alienation, abuse and rejection. Consequently, an understanding of social expectations was critical in making sense of the ways in which these young men operated within their social webs and of the social success that they did or did not enjoy.

Therefore, individuals, like these young men, "are" bodies and "have" bodies, they do not simply exist "in themselves" but become the subject of enterprise, interest and reflection. With this in mind, human bodies are more often then not perceived, understood and experienced as unfinished projects and works-in-progress, which are not merely influenced by social and physical relationships, but also constructed, underpinned by, intensified, changed and consumed by those relationships. Our experiences may be uniquely different but our journeys are often the same, influenced by the innumerable social messages, expectations and norms that many young men struggle with, often in an attempt to portray an acceptable, desirable and individualistic body schema.

## Implications and Recommendations

As the study progressed over several months, the young men interviewed became increasingly aware of the various discourses that operated within their social spaces and the effects that these had on their bodies', behaviours, practices and identities. This was alluded to in Jack's final comment: "hmmm I have to say...its actually been good doing this survey. Never thought about this stuff before". Consequently, their interpersonal skills of reflection, self-awareness and reflexivity were strengthened as a result of their awareness of the way that various social influences like magazines, the internet, social media, television, marketing and advertising campaigns influenced their perception the world, their bodies and the bodies of those that surrounded them.

Are you aware of the effects of your social environment on your body image and on the body practices that you engage in? Are the body practices that you engage in beneficial or harmful to your health and well-being? And do you use your body image to your advantage?

One major concern that arose from the testimonies was the use of anabolic steroids for aesthetic and beauty purposes. Whilst many young men like Rocco are aware of the potential side effects of steroid use, which is enough to prevent them from practising risky image-enhancing practices, as alluded to by Rocco: "I wouldn't do them because they age you and because the size doesn't maintain. It just sounds all too hard", there are many that participate in risky behaviour regardless. Jack and Joe openly discussed using various types of steroids and they perceived that it was common practice amongst other gym goers. Both young men were not worried about possible short-term and long-term effects of these illegal drugs, despite experiencing numerous side effects, and they perceived their use of anabolic steroids as "safe" and "manageable". This phenomenon suggests a significant social trend given the recent reports published by the Australian Sports Anti-Doping Authority of widespread drug use amongst many professional Australian athletes, coaches and sports scientists. Steroid use amongst American athletes is also common as was shown by Lance Armstrong and his teammates' revelations, which revealed that many American pro cyclists and indeed cyclists throughout the world engaged in drug use to ensure a place on the podium and to attract financial backing by investors. News stories have also reported that steroid use is common amongst other American sports including wrestling, boxing, gymnastics, and American football. However, performance-enhancing drugs are no longer limited to professional athletes, since many young men, and women, have used steroids in increasingly large numbers to improve their appearance. The American Center of Disease Control reports that 4.1% of young men from the age of 17 have used steroids to improve their appearance, despite 62% of young men knowing that steroids could be detrimental to their health. Furthermore, 41% of American youths also reported that they knew where to buy and obtain steroids from. From my own experiences I suggest that this is simply the tip of the iceberg, and that many young men, particularly aged between 18- 35, who attend their local gym have more then likely used steroids at some point in their young lives, especially in areas where a desirable body is perceived to increase your chances of acquiring sex, social acceptance, improving your careers prospects, and having a relationship. Consequently, further research is needed to investigate young men's attitudes towards appearance-enhancing drugs and the detriments or/and benefits of steroid use, in order to discover if steroid use can be used in a regulated and safe manner. If you are considering using steroids you should consult a doctor before doing so.

The insights revealed within my research raise issues about male body dysmorphia; many young men, like, Joe, Jack and Rocco, feel that they need to attain an 'aesthetic-muscular' physique in order to be perceived by themselves and others as attractive, healthy and fit. It is important that health teachers and professionals are aware of these issues, and have the skills and knowledge to educate adolescents about the various influences (e.g. popular culture and mass media) affecting the way that young men understand themselves and express themselves through their bodies. It is also important that health professionals disprove the myth, portrayed through popular culture, that certain "natural" somatotypes are perceived to be healthier than others (e.g. mesomorph/muscular verses ectomorph/skinny or endomorph/large build).

But does education really work? As stated above, 62% of 17-year-olds already understand that steroids can have a detrimental effect on their health and well-being. And many of the young men that I know who take steroids to create a better-looking body are well educated professionals - doctors, teachers, lawyers, psychologists and so on - but they still feel the need to take steroids in order to ensure a sense of self and social acceptance. So, perhaps as a society we would fare better if we focused on further research to investigate and establish whether steroids (used to enhance one's physical appearance) can be used in a way that does not put the organs and lives of many young men at risk. Or do we simply need to accept our bodies for what they are and realise that the pursuit of perfection is an unattainable goal?

Although attaining a muscular and perceived good-looking body was associated with feelings of pleasure and achievement, many men did not perceive the actual process of sculpting their bodies through exercise, dieting and other numerous techniques as enjoyable. Consequently, there is a role for health and physical education practitioners to play, focusing on the development of health, sport and fitness programs that emphasise the positive intrinsic benefits of living a healthy lifestyle. For example, experiences that promote friendship, enjoyment, confidence, skill acquisition, leadership, motivation, and the wide range of physiological benefits (e.g. improved respiratory, cardiovascular, immune, neurological, muscular and skeletal systems) that individuals can acquire as a result of a balanced healthy lifestyle. Young men and women should be encouraged to concentrate on process goals (e.g. the enjoyment of cooking and eating healthy foods, and exercising for 30-60 minutes per day), which lead to acquiring the healthy, fit body that so many of us desire. They may not end up looking like Hercules, but encouraging people to focus on intrinsic and process goals will ensure that people live healthier and happier lives.

Given the short lived lives of these young men, further research into their bodily and identity experiences throughout the rest of their lives (e.g. adulthood and old age) would give an insight into the various socio-psychological processes that occur during a person's life as they grow older. What is the physical and psychological relationship that men and women have with their bodies and how has it affected their health and well-being, in a holistic sense? What are the various tensions, struggles and experiences that they negotiate throughout their lives? Entertainer Michael Lucas states:

> *Through every stage of life there is pressure to stay in shape. In my teens, I felt too skinny. In my twenties, I wasn't built enough. Then I became busy running a company, so there was less time to go to the gym…Your twenties can be tragic and your forties can be fabulous. I was happier in my thirties than in my twenties and I look forward to being happier in my forties and beyond.*

His commentary suggests that some people may become less anxious about their body image as they grow older and learn to embrace their bodies just as they are. Perhaps as we grow older, many of us learn to mellow and not to take life as seriously as we once did during our youth. We learn to focus on the things that really matter, such as family, the community, helping others and pursuing a career.

## FROM OBSESSION TO ACCEPTANCE

So how do you prevent yourself from becoming too self-conscious and too pre-occupied about your body image - the way that you look? Here are 10 strategies that will increase your self-confidence and help you to develop a positive body image.

### Goal Setting

Whilst some of us are overly preoccupied with our appearance and struggle to overcome an addiction to making ourselves look good, there are others who couldn't care less. Some of us are just too caught up in the hustle and bustle of life, multitasking ourselves into oblivion as we attempt to stay on top of our monthly bills. Managing and maintaining our body is the last thing on our mind, consequently many of us simply let ourselves go, and worry about the consequences when it's too late.

However, as a friend once told me, if there is a will there is a way. If you want to manage your body effectively it is vital that you set exercise and nutrition goals, goals that are specific and that will hold you accountable. For example, you may set a goal of that completing 30 minutes of running/walking, six times a week, and of eating a healthy diet that contains a variety of fruits and vegetables, five to six times a day.

Ensure that you achieve your goals that you set goals that are realistic and challenging, yet attainable.

Set both short-term and long-term goals. Long-term goals provide information about your direction, whilst short-term goals enable you to monitor your progress towards your long-term goals. Short-term goals make your long-term goals more manageable, and increase your motivation as you achieve each short-term goal. As you achieve your short-term goals you will experience feelings of competency, skill mastery and accomplishment. To stay focused, write down your goals and display them in a place where you can see them on a frequent basis (e.g. your fridge). Writing goals down and displaying them in a prominent place will enable you to visualise your progress and consequently to increase your commitment, keeping you motivated as you move closer to your long-term goals.

## Stay in the Moment

Focus on staying in the 'moment' and enjoy the process of engaging in physical activity and eating healthy and nutritious food. Take pride in your body and praise yourself as you notice your body changing through committing yourself to a healthy lifestyle. Monitor your progress and record notes in a journal. How do you feel? How is your body changing? What physiological and psychological changes have you noticed? For example you may notice that you are stronger, have increased flexibility, improved breathing and sleep patterns, you may be less stressed, have lower cholesterol and blood pressure, and you may be happier and more confident with clearer skin and so on.

Be grateful for the body and mind that you have and use them to their full potential.

In moments of stress and anxiety concentrate on your breathing. Sit still, close your eyes, clear your mind and focus on the present. Slowly breathe in deeply through your nose and exhale out of your mouth. Repeat this process until you are totally relaxed. Focus on your technique, and let your body and mind relax.

## Be Intrinsically Motivated

Many fitness and beauty professionals and companies lure us into using their services and products with promises of body perfection, which will inevitably change our lives. For only $99.95 we'll look great, feel great, and live happily ever after. However, as many of us have already experienced, despite our best attempts, and despite spending a small fortune, our bodies still look the same. Feelings of hope turn into despair, emotions of guilt emerge and we blame ourselves for our inability to shape up. After a few months of trying, we quickly give up on our nutrition and fitness regimes because our bodies do not resemble the attractive bodies that we see in the media or on the sports fields.

And if you have managed to re-sculpt and change your body by spending hours in the gym, or by turning to cosmetic surgery, or by using drugs, it quickly becomes difficult to maintain this appearance.

Unfortunately, unless you have been genetically blessed with the body that you want to create, which is usually a lean (ectomorphic) or muscular (mesomorphic) physique, you won't be able to change your bone structure naturally, or dramatically change the amount of muscle - or even fat - that you are currently carrying. The genetic make-up of your body is predetermined from birth, and there is not much you can do about it.

The secret to developing and maintaining a positive attitude towards your own body image is to focus on the intrinsic benefits of engaging in healthy body practices like exercising and eating a nutritious diet. Involve yourself in physical activities that you enjoy and have fun with what you eat. If you don't enjoy training at the gym, participate in a physical activity that you do like. Join a walking or hiking group, or a sports club, or roll up your sleeves and create a beautiful vegetable garden for yourself. Experiment and try different foods and cuisines – Indian, Thai, Mediterranean, Japanese - and learn about the cultures from where the food originates. Creating a healthy lifestyle doesn't have to be a tedious chore.

Research shows that intrinsic motivation, participating in something because you enjoy it, is essential for maintaining adherence to long-term exercise and a healthy eating regime. The extrinsic rewards will take care of themselves. After six months of regular exercise and eating a healthy diet full of fresh fruit and vegetables you will notice improvements in your skin, your eyes, your cardio-vascular and cardio-respiratory health; you will notice decreased body fat and increased muscle mass, and you will begin to feel more confident as you begin to master new physical skills, movements, exercises and sports. You might not look like a supermodel, but you will be healthier. So embrace and accept the physique that you embody, make the most of it, and enjoy it!

## Remember...It's All An Illusion

When you find yourself looking through your favourite glossy magazine, as you admire the chiselled six-pack abs, the sexually desirable sculpted torso and the perfectly tanned silky smooth skin, remember that it's all an illusion. Great lighting, make-up, a professional photographer, and some nip and tuck tools courtesy of Photoshop can make anyone look good. Your favourite celebrity or model certainly doesn't look this perfect first thing in the morning when they wake up. The images, and the models that you find yourself admiring, which make many of us reflect upon our own bodies, and which at times make us feel self-conscious and anxious about our own physiques, have often been edited, airbrushed, manipulated, altered, retouched, refined and remastered. They aren't photographs as such, they are works of art.

## Choose Your Friends Wisely

Research shows that we are the sum of the five people that we spend most of our time with - our family, our friends, or our colleagues. It is therefore important that you surround yourself with people who are supportive, encouraging, and who have a positive 'can-do' attitude. Whether you are aware of it or not, your social network, you circle of friends influences your subconscious and conscious mind. Your social network significantly influences the way that you think and behave, what you think of yourself and what you think that you are capable of. Research suggests that if your friends and family believe in you, then you are more likely to achieve your goals, and you are more likely to see yourself in a positive light.

Consciously seek out friends and mentors that will give you the support and guidance that you need in order to achieve your goals. Surround yourself with people that lift you up, and avoid those who want to pull you down.

## *Be positive*

What we think and the way that we think of ourselves define not only who we are and what we do, but the type of person that we become. For many of us we become the person that we think we should be, and often the person that others expect us to be. We are a product of our conscious and subconscious minds, and we often reflect the cultural values and social expectations that we are immersed within. The key to reaching your full potential is to understand how our thoughts and social environments affect our self-perception and our progression through life. At some point in your life you may need to break free from these socially constructed truths, thoughts, and ideals in order to ensure that you create the life that you deserve.

The difference between success and failure is not influenced by your genetics, your appearance, who your friends are or even your IQ. Your success in life is determined by the degree that you believe in yourself. If you think you can - you will, but if you think you can't - you won't. Believe in yourself and go for it! Achieve the goals that you have set yourself and don't let self-doubt and a few roadblocks get in your way. Sure, some of us have higher mountains to climb, but don't let a few more layers of snow stop you from making the most of your ability. Surround yourself with good people, think highly of yourself, dare to dream, and take action.

Develop your confidence and self-image with positive affirmations. Tell yourself that you're beautiful, that you're talented, and that you will be successful. Be thankful for all of life's experiences, good and bad, and think of these experiences as lessons that are designed to increase your understanding of the world. When you perceive negative experiences as teachings that are designed as guidance, you are less likely to experience feelings of stress, anger and resentment, and you are more likely to take responsibility for your actions, achieve your life goals and have a positive perception of yourself and others.

You are what you think; if you think positive thoughts and truly believe in them you will become a positive person. Use positive affirmations to create your own reality. Why create a reality of doom and gloom with negative self-talk and self-defeating statements that you use to subconsciously sabotage your own life, when you can create a reality full of opportunities by being positive? Use positive affirmations to create the life that you deserve. Confident people know that they will be successful and they're usually right.

## Don't Compare Yourself to Others

Comparing yourself, your body, your career, and your life to somebody who seems to have it all will always leave you feeling a little insecure, envious and disheartened. In a fast-paced world where we have become accustomed to getting what we want - when we want it - we become easily frustrated when our desires are not achieved instantaneously. Instant gratification is not only demanded it's expected. Consequently, when we take on a new exercise regime or diet, in order to look like the world's next top super model, and our expectations aren't met within a short space of time, we either give up or turn to quick-fix solutions, which usually aren't good for us. Sometimes our desire to imitate someone else, someone more physically desirable, can lead to obsessive behaviour such as exercise or drug addiction, excessively weighing food, and counting every single calorie that goes into our mouths.

To maintain a healthy body and mind, it is important that you keep things in perspective. Trying to create and embody the physique of a professional athlete, bodybuilder, personal trainer, super model, or an actor who only works two months a year will always increase feelings of body anxiety, particularly if you work in an office nine to five. Be realistic when setting exercise and nutrition goals, and remember that your body type, i.e. your body's genetics, is unique to you and is unlikely to change drastically unless you engage in unhealthy body practices. Focus on creating a healthy body by eating a well-balanced diet and exercising regularly. Be patient, and focus on enjoying the moment. Focus too on the feelings of satisfaction and sense of achievement that you will experience when learning and developing new skills and creating a healthier body through eating a variety of nutritious foods and exercising regularly. Your body will naturally become healthier, stronger, faster, skilful, energetic, and more vibrant over time.

When choosing a sports club make sure the club's social and physical environment is welcoming, relaxed, and enjoyable. A sports club - particularly a gym - should be a place where you can unwind, relax and de-stress. Make use of free trial memberships to ensure that the club is right for you. If you are new to the gym scene you don't want to find yourself locked into a 12-month contract where you are surrounded by professional body builders whose biceps are bigger then your head, an intimidating environment that is likely to make you feel physically inadequate, self-conscious and overwhelmed. This may cause unnecessary stress and affect your self-confidence negatively. You are also more likely to engage in risky body practices (e.g. use steroids or obsess over food) to reflect the physiques that surround you, and to ensure - subconsciously and/or consciously - that you will be socially accepted by your new peers. To avoid feelings of being physically inadequate choose a gym where you feel that you belong, and not one where you feel out of your depth.

## You Are What You Eat

Have you ever wondered why some people are able to eat everything in sight yet never seem to put on any weight whilst others pile on the kilograms as soon as they look at a bowl of pasta or a freshly fried donut? How can someone eat like a horse and still manage to maintain a lean, healthy and well-defined body?

If you put on weight easily this is a question that you have probably asked yourself many times. You've tried every fad diet, various detox beverages, and purchased numerous exercise apparatuses that promise you a perfect body if you use them for five minutes every day, but the fat just won't melt away, and the muscles never appear.

Unfortunately, for millions of people around the world who struggle with their weight, despite their best attempts, they engage in unhealthy dieting practices when nothing else seems to work to ensure that they embody a socially desirable appearance. These unhealthy dieting practices may include restricting your food intake by eating only a few meals a day (or not eating at all), purging, fasting, binge-eating or obsessively monitoring everything that you eat. These unhealthy eating practices can quickly become habitual and lead to the onset of physical and psychological stress, obesity, diabetes, increased blood pressure, heart-disease and they predispose you to developing eating disorders such as anorexia and bulimia, which can have dire consequences for your health and well-being, i.e. death.

From my personal experience working with people who battle to keep their weight under control and who are dissatisfied with their body image, many of them either obsess over their body weight and how they are going to lose excess weight (whether they are overweight or not) or put on extra muscle, or they give up completely. These strategies are potentially hazardous and could impact the quality of your life significantly – your self-confidence, your perception of yourself, your attitude towards others, and your physiological health.

So how do you manage your body effectively and how can you create a healthy body? How do you become comfortable within your own skin and accept and love the physique that you have?

To prevent yourself from engaging in unhealthy eating habits and from experiencing feelings of body anxiety it is important that you understand the way your body reacts to different types of food.

Whilst some people's bodies metabolise food quickly - usually those with leaner physiques - there are many people who metabolise food at a slower rate, and they usually embody a naturally muscular or larger shape. The trick is to figure out if your body metabolises food quickly or slowly.

If your body expends energy easily and metabolises food quickly you will find that you are instinctively hungry; wanting to graze and eat throughout the day. This is perfectly normal for your body type (e.g. lean and/or athletic). To ensure that your body functions to its optimum and gets enough fuel (energy), it is important that you eat five or six small to regular sized meals (ideally the size of your hand) regularly, preferably every 2 to 3 hours, and consume a diet with plenty of carbohydrates (breads, grains, rice, pasta). You should also inckude vegetables, fruits, fish, meat, nuts and dairy products, and protein (meat, fish, eggs) in your diet. This will provide your body with enough sustenance, nutrients and energy to work effectively throughout the day. Those with a lean physique will find that they naturally find it difficult to put on weight and muscle, regardless of the amount they eat and exercise.

On the other hand, if you find that you put on weight easily, even when you don't eat, it is likely that you have a naturally muscular or larger body, and that you metabolise food slowly because you do not expend as much energy in a physiological sense. If this is the case, try eating three to four larger meals, the size of your hand, at regular intervals throughout the day, with snacks consisting of fruit, nuts, cheese, or even delicious fruit smoothies (if you are constantly on the go) in order to keep your mind and body focused from morning to night. Your body does not expend as much energy; therefore you don't have to eat as much or as regularly as those who possess a naturally leaner physique. Because your body naturally expends less energy performIing day-to-day tasks you do not need to consume as many carbohydrates, which are energy-dense. When someone with a larger physique consumes too many energy-rich foods (sugar, breads, rice, pasta), the excess energy (sugar) from the food eaten is stored within your body for later use. However, if this stored energy isn't utilised and expended through physical movement, soon afterwards the excess energy will be converted into fat eventually. Consequently, extra layers of fat slowly but surely begin to appear around your waist, thighs and buttocks. If you love eating pasta, bread, rice, or sugary foods, consume them in moderation during the day, when you need to make use of the energy that they give to your body, and focus on eating protein and vegetables for dinner - and eat clean!

"Eating clean" (inspired by Japanese and Mediterranean eating habits) is an eating philosophy practised by many athletes and health professionals. "Eating clean" is a philosophy requiring you to eat a diet that consists of naturally grown fresh foods such as fruits, vegetables, grains, meat, fish, nuts and healthy oils (e.g. olive oil). Foods to avoid include unnatural and processed foods, which contain artificial sweeteners, preservatives, colours and flavours.

Many large national and multinational food companies such as McDonald's and Coca Cola put these unnatural ingredients, additives, into their food products to cut down on costs, maintain freshness, add flavour, improve taste and prolong their shelf life. Unfortunately, research suggests that many of these additives cause allergies, behavioural problems, obesity, diabetes, diseased organs, cancer and premature death. Whilst some governments around the world have introduced food standards and regulations to prevent food companies from using many toxic ingredients, there are many countries that have not.

To ensure that you're consuming food that is good for you, read the ingredients label carefully in order to avoid foods that you are suspicious of. You are what you eat, so feed your engine with the best fuel that you can find.

## Overcome Your Fears

For many, attending a gym or sports club for the first time is an intimidating experience. You find yourself in a crowded room surrounded by fitness junkies who seem to know exactly what they're doing whilst you stand there dumbfounded, as you don't have a clue. You feel self-conscious, anxious and insecure, and you don't plan on coming back anytime soon. This was certainly my experience when I first attended a fitness club.

To overcome these feelings of inferiority, if you decide to take part in an unfamiliar activity, find a supportive friend who you can train with, or seek help from an exercise professional, like a personal trainer, in order to familiarise yourself with the techniques and the skills needed, until you feel confident that you can work out on your own. This will increase your autonomy as you have the freedom to set and achieve your own goals, without someone else's schedule restricting you - and it's free! This can result in increased feelings of competence, achievement success and an increase in intrinsic motivation. Working out with a personal trainer all the time can decrease your autonomy, and can result in a reliance on your PT to get you through your exercises.

Attending group fitness classes is a great option as you can choose the classes you're interested in at the times that suit you. Many gyms have a range of activities, from yoga to kick boxing and pole dancing, taught at beginner to advanced levels. Group activities also give you a wonderful opportunity to meet new people and make new friends.

## Reward Yourself

Reward yourself! After completing a short-term goal, for example completing 30 minutes of aerobic exercise (e.g. running, walking, playing sport), six times a week for four weeks, reward yourself by taking a weekend away with your partner, go on a shopping spree, watch the latest movie, socialise with friends or eat out at your favourite restaurant. A personal reward system will keep you motivated and increase your adherence to your exercise and nutrition program.

Use these 10 simple strategies to help you to manage your body effectively and to control feelings of body anxiety and stress. These strategies will help you to feel more at ease, and feel confident and comfortable with your own body, enabling you to live a healthy and happy life.

# FINAL THOUGHT

While the human body has often been explored, analysed and understood within the paradigms of socio-cultural space and time, the experiences of the human body have often been an 'absent presence'. The voices and personal stories of the young men within this research afford a nuanced understanding of the lives and experiences of these and other young men. The complex and multi-faceted social and physiological influences that consciously and subconsciously affect their body image, various body constructing techniques, practices and behaviours, anxieties, pleasures, sense of self, and health and well-being. However, sometimes we all need to listen to the wisdom of the voices within, and ignore the negative influences that surround us. Whilst many people over-emphasise the importance of our physical selves, our beautiful spirits within will be remembered; we need to pay attention to them.

*"Anybody pretending to be anything other then who you really are, you will never ever reach your personal potential. You cannot do it...Your intention rules your life and determines the outcome...I don't care how beautiful you are, one day your breasts are going to sag and your eyes are going to bag, and your not going to be as beautiful. It doesn't matter how much botox and how many times you get yourself pulled up, and how many hairdos, and how many make over's or what you do, you know it doesn't last.*

*You know it's just like the most beautiful flowering tree, everything passes in its time. It doesn't matter how much money you have, how much power you have, how high you sit on the Forbes list, how many times you make the most influential lists, all that changes, all of that changes. But what is real, what is lasting is who you are, and what you were meant to bring, what is the gift you were meant to give and nobody can take that away from you."*

– Oprah Winfrey

# CHAPTER SIX

# Q & A:
# Shaping up in the 21st Century

## WHAT IS BODY IMAGE?

The term 'body image' is found in the work of scholars hailing from a range of academic disciplines (e.g. psychology, sociology, psychiatry, philosophy, and anthropology). The Austrian neurologist, psychoanalyst and researcher Paul Schilder first defined the term 'body image' in 1935. Isidore Ziferstein, a professor in psychiatry from the University of Southern California notes:

*"Schilder combined Carl Wernicke's concept of the somatopsyche, Sir Henry Head's postural model of the body, and Freud's idea that the ego is primarily a body ego, to arrive to his own formulation of the fundamental role of the body image in man's relation to himself, to his fellow human beings, and to the world around him."*

By his defininition body image referred to a person's perception of the aesthetics and sexual attractiveness of his or her own body. Schilder suggested that body image is "the picture of our body which we form in our mind, that is to say the way in which our body appears to ourselves". Contemporary scholars have since expanded on Schilder's earlier definition of body image to include aspects of a person's feelings and emotions. Psychology Professor Sarah Grogan defines body image in the following way:

*"Body image relates to a person's perceptions, feelings and thoughts about his or her body, and is usually conceptualized as incorporating body size estimation, evaluation of body attractiveness and emotions associated with body shape and size."*

Throughout history, human society has placed great value on the beauty of the 'ideal' masculine male body, which has changed over time, to reflect the socio-historical contexts in which people live. The value attached to bodies has shifted from admiration and worship of the masculine, wise and authoritative bodies of biblical heroes like King David, to the muscular, strong and powerful Greek mythological and Olympic gods like Zeus; to Hitler's pursuit of the ideal 'pure', 'Aryan' (Nordic) master race to the modern day adoration of well groomed and styled, beautiful celebrity bodies like those of David Beckham and Brad Pitt. These examples demonstrate that throughout history there have been bodies that have been portrayed as ideal; ideal bodies that many young men have tried to live up to them and aspired to achieve them. Admiration of these desirable bodies is reflected in statues and paintings, and also within the mass media, on television and throughout social media. All these representations serve to reinforce and construct a definition of the 'ideal' male body. These male bodies are often celebrated, worshiped and admired because they represent status, success, wealth, power, athleticism, intelligence, masculinity and beauty. Consequently, many young men and women, consciously and subconsciously, will do whatever it takes to embody these desirable characteristics by creating an appealing physical appearance in order to feel accepted within the communities that they live.

Both psychological and sociological research has suggested that a person's body image contributes to his or her personal experiences and personality, and plays a major role in the construction of their personal identity. For example, research with adolescents and young men, found that populations of youth were constantly self-checking, and were self-conscious of any aspect of their body that might be stigmatised, thus leading to harassment and embarrassment in front of their peers. Psychological studies that interviewed young men throughout the western world found that:

> "...being lean and muscular was linked to being healthy and fit. Being fat was related to weakness of will and lack of control... Sixteen-year-olds described peer pressure to be slender and muscular, and two young men had experienced teasing about their body size. ...teenagers explicitly linked having a well-toned, muscular body with feelings of confidence and power in social situations."

These discourses suggest that many young men feel pressured to create and maintain a socially accepted body, usually a body devoid of excessive fat or muscle, in order to avoid being alienated and harassed by their peers. The socially accepted and desirable taught muscular body is attributed to feeling healthy, confident, powerful and strong whilst a fat body often leaves young men feeling unhealthy, weak and inferior; it evokes a loss of physical and psychological control.

Culture, gender, sexual orientation and social class inevitably contour one's body image. So too do body ideals that are cultivated and transmitted by social and mainstream media. As alluded to in chapter one, since the 1980's images of the 'ideal' lean, muscular and handsome male body have increased within the mass advertising media. However, unlike the 1980's, advertising is not restricted to our televisions, the occasional billboard and women's magazines. The 'ideal' male body is presented to us via television, glossy men's lifestyle magazines, social media (e.g. Youtube, Facebook and Instagram), online press media and personal emails. We are surrounded by images of the 'ideal' 'aesthetic-athletic' male body 24 hours a day! It is therefore, not surprising that this dramatic increase in the presentation of the 'ideal' youthful, handsome, athletically shaped male physique, through new technologies and contemporary forms of social media, is increasingly effecting - for better or worse - the way that young men perceive their bodies and the way they think their bodies should look.

While one might imagine that focusing on one's own body shape, comparing it to media images and so on, might yield a fairly accurate assessment of body shape, size and appearance, research to date suggests that a distorted rather than a realistic body image is the norm for many young people. Harvard professor of psychiatry Harrison Pope suggests that many young men regard themselves as larger or smaller than they actually are – a phenomenon which could lead to psychological and health issues such as body anxiety, anorexia, bulimia, exercise addiction or muscle dysmorphia. Australian research into body image among adolescents over the past four decades has shown a continual progression towards a more distorted and negative perception of the body, despite most adolescents being of a normal body weight. Furthermore, research throughout the United States, Europe and Australia suggests that young men's attitudes reflect a desire for 'bigness', muscularity, strength and masculinity. So what are the social influences that are leading young men to have 'distorted' perceptions of their own bodies within the world they live?

Young men are currently growing up in an era of high modernity, an era where one's physical, and even virtual identity and body is created, structured and influenced through the values of capitalism, individualism, the consumption of materialistic goods, the freedom of individual choice and constant self-surveillance in order to ensure that one is of good health and that we are contributing to the economy. The increased scrutiny and pressure placed upon many young males from a variety of perspectives including popular culture, peers, and societal and cultural expectations, often without them realizing it, to create and present a modern 21st century archetypal male body has seen a dramatic increase in the number of young males with body image issues over the past 15 to 20 years.

## WHAT IS MASCULINITY?

The primary theme that arises from the practices and behaviours of young men in relation to their body image is the desire to embody physical, emotional and psychological practices associated with 'manliness'. According to many sociologists in the western world the most desirable characteristics that boys want to portray are physical strength, competency through sport, an athletic or muscular body, 'toughness' and the restraint of one's emotions in order to eliminate supposed emotional weaknesses such as crying. Sociologist Raewyn Connell defines masculinity as:

> *"Masculinity is a pattern of practice. So it's not an attitude, it's not what's in peoples' heads, it's not the state of their hormones, it's what they actually do in the world. ...It has a relationship to your body and biology but not a fixed relationship. So women can behave in a masculine way, though usually it's men who do, and also there are different patterns of masculinity. So different groups of men will conduct themselves in different ways and those patterns also can change over time.....some patterns of masculinity do include a willingness to use violence.... where other patterns of masculinity are in comparison peaceable."*

Sociological research suggests that gender roles, masculinity and femininity are learnt through individuals' engagement with society. Australian sport sociologist Richard Light states: "the learning of gender is different to common sense perceptions of learning as a rational, intellectual process. It is, instead, a long term, whole body, social process operating at a non conscious level making it implicit and difficult to understand". Throughout their school years, young boys' gender identities, attributes and desires are channeled and shaped through sport and physical education where clear distinctions between what it means to be masculine and feminine are made. Boys are taught masculinity traits like sportsmanship, competitiveness, the hunger and desire to succeed, toughness, aggressiveness, discipline, comradeship, physical skills and strength, and constructing strong masculine bodies through competitive sports, especially within private schools.

Men and boys conduct themselves in different ways. This may of course, change over time and vary within cultural, racialised, class, and religious contexts, but the hierarchical relationship of masculinities is based on the pattern of male practice and behaviour that is most valued and respected within a particular cultural setting. The dominant masculinity is the honoured masculinity, the leader of the pack, who is seen to have authority, power and dominance over other less honoured male masculinities who are often marginalized or even excluded within the society they live because they do not live up to the 'ideal' man. The dominant masculinity does not refer to a singular dominant male ideal, but multiple masculinities that have a hierarchical relationship with each other. Connell suggests that the dominant masculinity was not assumed to be normal in the statistical sense; only a minority of men might enact it. But it was certainly normative. It embodied the currently most honoured way of being a man and required all other men to position themselves in relation to it.

The relationship of masculinities within a hierarchical system is evident within the school environment. Dominant masculinities will compete against each other for power, prestige and status while more subordinate masculinities will be dominated, alienated and often bullied, whether it be in the corporate world, in tribal groups or in the school yard. Majella McSharry, an Irish sociology and education researcher found that the masculine identities that are validated and have power within the school system are those that are successful in sport and academia, being physically strong, athletic, sexually attractive, and having heterosexual partners. Her research suggests that there are five levels of validation that enable status and prestige.

1. Involvement in sport
2. Naturally smart and intelligent, but not a geek
3. Physical ability and performance in sport
4. Possessing a muscular/athletic body type
5. Having an active social life

So the handsome, naturally intelligent, gifted young male football player that embodies a muscular, athletic body and socialises with his girlfriend whilst partying at the weekend would be 'top dog' in the hierarchical tree of masculinity within, and even outside of, the confines of the school gates. Boys and young men that successfully participate in sport receive prestige, power and a higher social status within the school and they are recognised with trophies, awards, medals, sports jackets and an increase in popularity with their peers. These learned masculine practices and experiences engendered through school sport and reinforced through positive acknowledgements and rewards, are a pivotal influence on boys' gendered identities.

Boys that were highly 'validated' within the secondary school setting often used their power and status to demote and intimidate students who were less validated in order to maintain and increase their own social image and position within the school. Boys that were victimised due to their lack of masculinity, physical skill and appearance were labeled 'wimpy', 'fat', 'girly', 'stupid', 'unnatural', 'abnormal', 'gay', 'nerd' and 'unattractive', and were often left feeling rejected, alienated and powerless within the school. Students reported instances of self-harm, physical and emotional scars, decreased self-esteem and confidence, shame and personal failure because they did not meet the criteria of the 'ideal' male and because of their consequent low social status within the school. Of course, these social practices are not restricted within the school/college gates. Young men continue to use their physical capital within the office, the boardroom, the nightclub and anywhere else where it may be of benefit.

Consequently, young men are under enormous pressure from an early age to display masculine traits demonstrated by the dominant masculinities within their social environments in order to avoid being rejected, bullied and stigmatised. In some instances young men are taking extreme measures to create a more masculine body through risky diet and exercise regimes, buying costly sports supplements and even participating in drug use to ensure that they have a body that is socially accepted, in order to receive a higher social status and to distance themselves from being alienated and disowned by their peers.

## WHY HAVE WE BECOME SO PREOCCUPIED ABOUT THE PHYSICAL APPEARANCE OF OUR BODIES?

Throughout our social environment there are a variety of discourses and attitudes (e.g. medical, health, fitness, beauty and commercial) that inform our understanding of the various characteristics (e.g. masculine, strong, muscular, fit, healthy) and purposes (e.g. economic production, sport, relationships, physical defence – including war and a healthy lifestyle) of the 'perfect', 'normative' male (or female) body that one is encouraged to obtain, particularly through medical, and educational advice, and through corporations and government institutions. Ultimately, these discourses combine to define and position our bodies as winners or losers, acceptable or not acceptable, and to determine the abilities and subjectivities that will be recognised and celebrated – or not. These social messages impact on the way in which we view our own body and the bodies of others; they frame our understanding of 'what it is to be healthy' and what a healthy body looks like. However, these discourses often change over time due to shifting developments and understandings of knowledge acquired from medical, health and sports science research, which is communicated to us through the media, and through corporate and government organisations within our communities. In essence, for many of us, our subconscious mind is socially conditioned to create and obtain a physique that is perceived to be desirable.

Prior to the 1950s the body was positioned as an object in need of correction in order to compensate for the pathological failings of social class, family and home. Governments sought to correct young bodies through school physical education lessons.

*"Schools [placed an] emphasis on hygiene, wholesome diet and physical activity (Swedish gymnastics)...[focused] upon correcting the physical defects born of poverty, poor physical environment, diet and nutrition amongst the mass of working-class children newly found in city schools."*

Furthermore, physical education, within schools throughout the world in the early 1950s were motivated by a need for physical training and fitness in readiness for possible military action in order to protect the British Empire. To some extent these practices are still performed, particularly within Asia and the Middle Eastern countries where the threat of war is constant. This position flowed into the 1960s, and was labelled the 'Corrective' era of the body, informed by medico-health discourse. Similar to the time before the 1950s, "its focus is the body of deficit and in need of treatment and repair through compensatory intervention (e.g. via better hygiene, diet and healthy exercise)" (Evans & Davies). Schools continued to focus on the body as an 'imperfect' object generated through the circumstances of one's class; through poverty and self-neglect. The body was in need of being corrected, disciplined and controlled in preparation for an efficient and effective workforce.

In the 1970s work on the body was seen as 'ameliorative' and 'therapeutic', informed by the discourses of scientific functionalism and by the clinical and physical sciences, with the focus on improving the body through systems of training and exercise for health. School-based physical education focused on changing and improving young bodies through circuit training, fitness through sport and through improvements in diet as means of physical therapy to address the unsatisfactory standards of health in children and adolescents.

Therefore, not only did the body need to be corrected and controlled, as in the 1950s and 1960s, it also had to be improved upon. The body was treated as an unfinished machine in need of attention and care. It needed to be well oiled, maintained and ready for the production line of an ever increasingly Westernised capitalist society. Sport Sociologist James Cameron states:

> "The very nature of physical education and sport reveals the relations of power being played out in the body ... in keeping with a capitalist mode of production, sport bodies are disciplined through work: 'work out', 'speed work' etc... The body is thus subordinate to the purpose of physical education and sport. On the other hand, physical education and sport builds healthy bodies, it is also used to foster control over the mind."

This emphasis on producing mass young bodies as well maintained, refined, and disciplined machines, cultivated through school physical education and sport, in order to increase society's industrial and economic output, started to burn out in the western world by the end of the 1970s due to advancements in technology and the declining use of physical labour.

Since the 1980s, health discourses within the education, medical, health, media and political spheres have moved in a new direction. Health and well-being have since been both influenced and defined by both the physical and social sciences within medicine, health and sports science (e.g. physiology, biomechanics, psychology and sociology). There has been an increased emphasis on epidemiology and genetics, both inside and outside of the classroom, focused on "prevention through health promotion and intervention that is self-referential, dedicated to mind-set and lifestyle changes to diet, exercise and the avoidance of risk factors of modern society" (Evans & Davies). Consequently, young people have been taught to have an increased awareness of taking care of their bodies, reinforced by an increase in public health promotion, which has been communicated predominantly through schools and government advertising.

Discourses of the body have and are shaping the way that young men view, construct and understand their bodies, particularly through their participation in school physical education lessons. Reflecting upon health discourses within schools, Education professors Evans & Davies state:

> ....although there are tensions between the variety of health discourses and modalities now found in schools, all, in one way or another, focus on the body as imperfect (whether through circumstances of ones class and poverty, or self-neglect), unfinished and to be ameliorated through physical therapy (circuit training, fitness through sport and a better diet), threatened (by the risks of modernity/lifestyles of food, overeating, inactivity) and, therefore, in need of care and being changed.

Consequently, it should be of no surprise that many young men feel anxious about their bodies. Young men have been taught through their schooling experiences and through the health discourses privileged in school physical education curriculums that their bodies are imperfect, unfinished, threatened and in need of being worked upon and changed in order to be healthy. Young men are not taught to accept and embrace their bodies as living, breathing, enjoyable organisms. Instead their bodies are often reduced to machines that are in need of consistent monitoring and management in order to ensure that they are healthy and that they are contributing to society. And let's not forget, while there are those who take to the gyms and sporting activities like ducks to water, there are also many young men who quickly give up on their bodies once they break down, run out of steam and once they become in need of repair, thus falling into psychological and physical despair, disheartenment, and losing hope of ever creating the healthy perfect body they are taught to desire. Sports historian Douglas Booth argues, "Humans unquestionably derive pleasurable physical sensations from different types of movement. Yet, remarkably, there is a deafening silence around the subject in the literature on human movement". For example, pleasures in rugby or football are derived from the sense of mock battle, friendships and teamwork, from development and displays of skill, fitness and strategy, and from physical contact and intimacy. Experiences of pleasure may also encompass a heightened awareness of the senses, fro example equilibrioception (balancing on precipices) and kinesthesia (the slow, deliberate movements of tai chi) and emotions associated with positive social relationships.

Thus young men are not taught to embrace their natural bodies as physical, social, spiritual, intellectual and pleasurable beings through the healthy practices of human movement. These movements include exercise, nutrition, socialising, friendship, work/life balance, contribution to society and so on, within and outside of school physical education. Consequently, due to a lack of perceived pleasure, many young men equate good health to shaping up and attaining six-pack abdominals, accompanied with large muscular biceps and pectorals. I argue that if young men were taught to be more accepting and embracing of their naturally existing bodies and identities, they would be more likely to participate in healthy habits, thus easing their anxiety about the way that their bodies should appear and behave.

A major concern about young men's bodies within research throughout the world over the last 10 years is the burgeoning evidence of young men's dissatisfaction with their bodies. Discourses of perfection are influencing the way that young men perceive their bodies, exacerbated by the incorporation of these modes within school-based physical education and sporting practices, and within the mass media. Many young men feel that their bodies are not accepted within the world that they live and often take extreme measures including drug use, cosmetic surgery and constant self-analysis in order to live up to western society's ideal image of a masculine, heterosexual, 'aesthetic-athletic', productive machine.

Numerous sociology and psychology research studies investigating young gay men's experiences of their bodies, including those involving participants in Australia, the United States of America, Canada and the United Kingdom report body dissatisfaction. These studies found that young gay men were often rejected, victimised and taunted by their peers, and even teachers, for embodying an identity and body that did not reflect the 'norm' of a masculine, athletic male body. These studies found that many young men sought ways of becoming more 'masculine' by physically reconstructing their bodies through strict eating regimes, weight lifting, cardiovascular exercise and steroid use in order to either lose weight (fat) or increase weight (muscle) so that they could meet the bodily prerequisites of an ideal and normative male physique. Many gay young men and heterosexual men who exhibited perceived feminine characteristics reported low levels of self-esteem, and confidence, often disowning their bodies and identities as they struggled for acceptance. This is reflected within the popular English gay magazine 'Attitude' as two gay male adolescents give an insight into their lives:

> I'm 15, still at school and it's a living hell. People trip me up and call me names and there's no one I can tell. My parents hate gays. I told my RE [Religious Education] teacher, but he treats me like I'm ill. I feel like a stranger at school, like in a freak show. Why can't I be treated normally? (Chris, 15)

> I'm very depressed and very alone... I used to be a perfect pupil getting high credit marks, but because of the bullying my marks have fallen to a foundation level. I can't tell anyone. I wish I was dead – just to have some peace. I am so tired of this so-called life... (Anon, 17).

Acknowledging the experiences of young gay men and their relationship with their bodies is important, as many may display characteristics and behaviours not associated with the 'normative' and 'desirable' heterosexual masculine body as alluded to by Rocco and

Joe. Although there are many young gay men who do display these desirable 'manly' traits and who embody the 'right' body and identity that may enable them to escape the judgements and scrutiny of the public eye because they do not display characteristics of a stereotypical gay identity, there are many who do not. I would also like to point out that these experiences are not only restricted to young gay men, as any young man who does not represent the ideal body image within their socio-cultural space maybe subjected to the same alienating experiences.

Furthermore, Australian Professor Murray Drummond, a specialist in men's body image, sought to explore and uncover the cultural myth that gay men are more susceptible to body image concerns due to the aesthetic-oriented gay culture. Participants in his study made the following comments in regards to their personal experiences and their observations of other young gay men's bodies and identities:

> "Men are supposed to be strong physically. They are supposed to be able to lift those incredible weights. I guess it's associated with virility. If someone is strong they're going to be virile."

> "For me, this image (of the muscular male) is of someone being in control, cool, calm, collected, or whatever."

> "....in certain parts of my life, I have to act a certain way just to fit in, to fit into certain communities. For instance if I go to Uni, I will sort of act slightly different and wear slightly different things than if I go to a gay club. Like, when I'm at Uni I won't expose a lot, you know. Like, I just wear normal Uni clothes. I use my glasses as a disguise when I want to look studious....I also have friends like that too who go to Uni and the Venus bar. They're two different places."

These comments emphasise the need for gay men to embody identities that reinforce the societal expectations of men to portray a desirable normative 'manly' persona, particularly when they are in social and public settings, where all eyes are focused on their every move in order to ensure that they conduct themselves 'appropriately'. However, as alluded to in the last comment and within Rocco, Joe's and Jack's statements, gay men often portray multiple identities, behaviours and social practices depending on the environment they are socialising in. They display more masculine traits in common spaces such as a university campus, as opposed to presenting their bodies in a more desirable way - with possibly less masculinity - or presenting their 'natural' selves in a gay club. Drummond goes on to highlight further findings from his research by saying:

> "....the influx of gay males into the bodybuilding subculture was largely a consequence of not wanting to look thin and unhealthy in the wake of the cultural HIV/AIDS panic. By maintaining a slender physique that had been stereotypically linked to gay men, there was a possibility of being perceived as having contracted HIV/AIDS. Therefore, as a form of protest muscularity, gay men began entering gyms to develop size and musculature."

Critically, this comment demonstrates the role of 'intervention, prevention and health promotion' health discourses hat are communicated to young men and the general pubic within their social webs, because individuals have been encouraged to take care of their own health and well-being in an effort to avoid ill health ever since the 1980s. One must avoid ill health, and also avoid displaying the characteristics of ill health at all costs in order to be considered as a healthy and productive citizen. This need for young gay men (and arguably 'straight' men) to obtain a healthy, sexually 'virile', muscular, masculine, attractive physique is reinforced through the various provocative images of men within gay media.

Sociologists Tate and George describe this phenomenon of sexually provocative images bombarding the minds of young gay men as "the toxic effects of the commercial gay scene", images which emphasise highly athletic muscular physique[s] - devoid of fat and hair, and usually clothes. This 'intoxication' of, a (at times unachievable) desirable youthful, muscular, aesthetically pleasing body, arguably affects the identities and the bodies that many young men want to acquire in order to be seen as attractive, wanted and accepted by others within the gay community.

The multiple discourses that currently reside within young men's social networks, particularly within the western world, are all intentionally or/and inadvertently encouraging young men to think of their bodies as imperfect, unfinished, threatened and in need of change. These discourses are articulated through national curriculums and teachers, health professionals, television, mass media, the internet, friends and family or businesses out to sell you the latest body shaping fad.

## WHAT IS A HEALHTY BODY?

A person's perceptions and experiences of his/her body can be understood further by examining the concept of 'healthism'. 'Healthism' as a set of beliefs that combines the "public objectives for the good health and good order of the social body with the desire of individuals for health and well-being". The emphasis on preventative health since the 1980s has lead to the emergence of 'healthism', a term describing ideological concerns of health and well-being where the individual is rendered responsible for the prevention and management of disease. 'Healthism' was a term born out of American politics, and used as a tool by governments during the 1970s to establish and impose norms of health.

An ideology of healthism states that disease or poor health is caused by unhealthy behaviours and practices, through poor self-management, too many cream pies, alcohol, tobacco, late nights, 'tube' watching, drugs, sex and rock 'n' roll, and of course a lack of physical activity. Consequently, the burden of remaining healthy is no longer on the shoulders of the government. Rather, the individual - i.e. you - are accountable for your own bodily health.

'Healthism' has influenced the rise of young men pursuing body perfection, because commercial enterprises, driven by business interests and profits, look to prey upon the health insecurities of potential customers. Over the last 20 years the health and fitness industry has become a multi-billion dollar industry with promises of longevity, encouraging us to stay healthy, and to engage in body redesign, with underlying discourses of obesity and self-starvation fueling this quest. The need for young men to self-manage and control their body image through becoming fit, active, muscular, masculine and healthy is reinforced by government and commercial networks, for example, American government health prevention campaigns like 'Lets Move' and 'Don't get smacked by FAT: Calories from sugary drinks can cause obesity and Type II diabetes which reinforces the need for regular exercise and a healthy diet in order to maintain a healthy body and lifestyle.

While many academics and members of society have cynically viewed 'healthism' as a coercive political tool, others have embraced the new opportunities that 'healthism' has created in the 21st Century. In the last 20 years, access to sports, health and fitness centres, and health practitioners has increased throughout the Western world making it easier to participate in preventative health; sponsoring fun, new, exciting exercise fads and trends of health to enjoy. These newfound health and fitness developments have encouraged young men to live a healthy lifestyle and manage their bodies independently. Furthermore, to some extent, government health campaigns throughout the world may be working. Statistical analysis suggests that obesity amongst

American children has slightly decreased, whilst obesity amongst adults has stabilised. However, obesity amongst older Americans over 60, continues to rise.

The research investigating young men's understanding of health and the impact their understandings have on their bodies has revealed a number of trends in relation to young people's gender roles - what a healthy body is and what it looks like. In response to the research question: "How do you know if a person is healthy? Many adolescents suggested that evaluating health was simply a matter of 'looking' at a person, assessing their size, shape, (and/or assessing their eating and exercise behaviours) and making judgments about their weight. These findings cohere with the results of several studies of adolescents' knowledge and understanding of health drawn from youth populations in Canada, Australia, Europe, and the United States, suggesting that young people predominantly conceive healthy living as a matter of eating and exercising, which is reflected in one's body shape. These research results also highlight an apparent lack of an understanding of more holistic versions of health and well-being that incorporate and support the development of social, spiritual, emotional and mental dimensions of health, despite these dimensions being part of many national physical education and health curriculums.

The 'healthism' discourses reinforced through the various social establishments encourage young men - and the rest of society - to take responsibility for their own health and well-being. This process, influenced by government and commercial organisations and agendas, often focuses on extrinsic benefits (e.g. looking good) in order to maintain a healthy population as opposed to a holistic approach that incorporates the care of one's total health and well-being. Consequently, the emphasis placed on creating the perfect physique, via popular culture, encourages many young men to think that good health is restricted to the 'aesthetic-athletic' body type. Those who do not measure up to these normative ideals are usually perceived as fat, skinny and/or unhealthy. To overcome feelings of physical inadequacy it is important for young men and women to understand that being healthy is not only reflected in your appearance, it is a reflected in the way that you think, your thoughts, your behaviour, the way that you treat and interact with others, your spirit, your intelligence, your confidence and the contribution that you make to your community and indeed the world. These are all measures that determine the true level of your health.

## WHAT IS BODY SURVEILANCE?

More then ever, throughout history, our bodies are being placed under constant surveillance and scrutiny through the various public and private sector lenses that monitor an individual's behaviour within the social spaces they inhabit. As signalled earlier, no public space - or even private space - is free from bodily surveillance. Images of our every movement are snapped using modern technology and placed on public display. People's bodies can be showcased and judged through social networking forums, television and print media throughout the world within seconds. The human body is constantly being analysed, policed, managed, governed, accepted and rejected by the world we live in.

Contemporary sociologist David Lyon defines surveillance as the monitoring of behaviour and activities - usually of people - for the purpose of influencing, managing, directing and protecting. Governments and law enforcement organisations use public surveillance to maintain social control, to recognise and monitor threats, to prevent and investigate criminal activity, and to monitor the progress of health and disease within a community. Together with several contemporary scholars, I argue that there are various reasons why there has been an increased and intensified level of surveillance of one's body and identity, within the western world in the last 15 years. Firstly, society's awareness and attempts to guard against terrorism have been heightened significantly since the 9/11 attacks in the

United States of America. Secondly, the rise of the obesity epidemic has increased people's awareness of their personal health and the need to take preventative measures, such as maintaining a healthy diet and regular exercise in order to ensure that they do not fall victim to cardiovascular and other preventable diseases (e.g. Type II diabetes). Thirdly, the increased power and ability of the mass media to record and publish highly confidential images and telephone messages of high profile political and government officials, and celebrity figures - as demonstrated by the media tycoon Rupert Murdoch's press scandal in 2011 - demonstrates that even those individuals who are well-guarded from the media are not protected from the constant surveillance that surrounds them. Many civil rights and privacy groups, such as the National Council for Civil Liberties (United Kingdom) and the American Civil Liberties Union, have expressed concern that by allowing continual increases in citizen surveillance we will end up in a mass surveillance society, with extremely limited, or non-existent political and/or personal freedoms, along with limited freedom to express ourselves freely. Every move, action and decision we make will be analysed and scrutinised by governments, friends, family and complete strangers. The potential dangers of mass surveillance were realised when former national security agent Edward Snowden infamously blew the whistle on the United States government organisation the NSA (National Security Agency) for illegally spying and collecting private information on its citizens. In an interview with The Guardian, a British newspaper, Edward Snowden states:

> *"You've got young enlisted guys, 18 to 22 years old, they have suddenly been thrust into a position of extraordinary responsibility where they now have access to all of your private records. Now in the course of their daily work, they stumble across something that is completely unrelated to their work in any sense. For example, an intimate nude photo of someone in a sexually compromising situation, but they're extremely attractive. So what do they do? They turn around and they show their coworker. And their coworker says 'Oh hey, that's great. Show it to Bill down the*

*way.' And then Bill sends it to George, George sends it to Tom, and sooner or later this person's whole life has been seen by all of these other people. It's never reported, no one ever knows about it because the auditing of these systems is incredibly weak....[It's] a violation of your rights."*

Furthermore, in a CNN interview Snowden states:

*"...all of our data can be collected without any suspicion of wrong doing on our part, without any underlying justification. All your private communications, all of your private communications, all of your transactions, all of your associations, who you talk to, who you love, what you buy, what you read. All of these things can be seized and held by the government and then searched later for any reason, without any justification, without any real oversight, without any real accountability for those who do wrong."*

Whilst many believe that this mass surveillance is necessary in order to keep us safe from the potential threats of terrorism, and that the only people who should be concerned are those who have done something wrong, this appears to be wishful thinking. The ability for governments to access your personal records – photos, emails and videos - could be taken out of context and used against you, particularly if you have information that puts the government's political capital in jeopardy. This was revealed to me when an older friend of mine discussed his mother's experience of living in Germany during World War II. She believed that she was safe from Hitler's pursuit of world domination and had nothing to fear as she embodied what Hitler was looking for – at least physically. She told her son: "They went after the Jews, they went after refugees, they went after the intellectuals, they went after the writers and journalists, they went after the children, but then they came for me." When governments - and those associated with the government (i.e. the armed forces) - abuse their powers, we should all be worried and consequently do our upmost in order to ensure that our civil liberties and freedoms are secure. Although we may try our best to shape up and create a desirable identity - to live up to the social norms and expectations that surround us and thus avoid unwanted suspicion, sometimes it's still not good enough for the powers that be.

In the last five years, scholars and investigative journalists have reported the emergence and rise of racial profiling, whereby police deliberately target ethnic minorities (e.g. African-Americans) in order to reduce crime. American, British, Australian and New Zealand social research clearly shows that ethnic minorities are more likely to be dealt with brutally, accused and arrested for criminal activity, and sometimes killed because of the colour of their skin, even when they have done nothing wrong. However, instances of bigotry and discrimination are not only limited to specific ethnicities. People are often discriminated against and taken at face value because of their social class, hair colour, age, body type, political bias, sexuality, career, interests, dress sense and so on. From young people wearing hoodies, to people of colour; from the homeless to a Wall Street banker, or a retiree; at some point in our lives, many of us have been victims of bigotry because of the way we look.

Whether we realise it or not, we are all typecast and stereotyped into specific identities – the ditzy blonde, the dumb jock, the lazy obese, the selfish capitalist, the Muslim extremist, the abnormal queer, the stupid African-American and the greedy rich are all identities which are used to label specific groups of people. These stereotypes - often misleading - influence and shape our subconscious minds and the way we think about and interact with others. Socially constructed stereotypes - which are usually created in order to alienate and disempower groups of people - affect our perception of others and of their capabilities, our selection of employees and employers, the people whom we avoid, whom we spend time with and often whom we marry. So, next time you find yourself making a judgment about somebody you see on the other side of the street or on television whom you have never met; stop and think about the reason for your judgement. How can you judge somebody whom you have never met? What has influenced your perceptions of this person and where do these perceptions come from? As a wise man once said – "you should never judge a book by its cover", you'll be pleasantly surprised by most people's content and the life stories that they have to tell.

## Surveillance of the Self

Sociologist John Hargreaves argues that social surveillance is an ideal method for controlling modern consumer-based societies. He points out that self-surveillance - reinforced by government policies (e.g. health, law and order, and education) and the mass media - is an effective way of enforcing acceptable levels of bodily control, discipline, appearance and behaviour of individuals within a society.

> *"Our increased visibility to each other in public - street, work, office, school, college, media, beach, health club - constitutes a comprehensive system of mutual discipline far more relentless than repressive discipline. Witness the disciplined enjoyment of freely chosen activities like jogging, dieting, dressing fashionably, keeping clean, applying unguents and cosmetics, playing sports, displaying at discos, and consider the volume of freely chosen goods and services consumed in the process of producing oneself as the youthful, authentic man or woman."*

Prominent sociologist Michel Foucault refers to the bodily practices and behaviours that individuals police, monitor and maintain in respect to their own bodies as 'Technologies of Self'. One of the main features of technologies of self is the relationship between scientific expertise and self-regulation which are implicit within these technologies. Expertise is grounded within the authority of scientific and objective truth established by the medical research of universities and other government institutions. Information regarding one's personal health, one's body and how to take care of it, is grounded and supported by this medical and scientific truth, which is then introduced and 'mobilised' through government establishments such as schools and health agencies. It is also reinforced by public health media campaigns and propaganda. All of these processes encourage individuals to take on healthy practices and behaviours that will ostensibly increase the quality of their lives. Consequently, individuals - sometimes inadvertently - self-regulate their bodies into healthy shapes and sizes based on the knowledge and expertise imputed on them via their surrounding medical and health discourse. Expertise works through a logic of choice, "inculcating desires for self-development that expertise itself can guide and through claims to be able to allay the anxieties generated when the actuality of life fails to live up to its image" (Rose). In an attempt to 'shape up' and take responsibility for our personal health and well-being, individuals pursue practices of the technologies of the self, including going to the gym, following fad diets, quick fix remedies and electronic monitoring devices ('the quantified self'). These devices measure everything from your sleep patterns to your blood pressure and the number of calories that you burn every day, and indeed anything else that will put your health and body anxieties at ease as you attempt to avoid being 'out of shape' and unhealthy. Innovations in various technologies such as iphone applications have been of benefit and are enjoyed by many that use them, as they allow the user to keep a close eye on body fat, sugar intake, body weight, sleeping patterns and so on. For many others, use of these applications may lead to an unhealthy preoccupation and an obsession with one's bodily appearance.

## Surveillance Medicine

It is not as if examination and surveillance are new events or processes. Throughout history bodies have always been subjected to medical and/or public examination, as young men (and the rest of society) grow up being analysed, poked and prodded in the pursuit of a diagnosis (i.e. the 'mad', 'bad', 'good', 'guilty', 'ugly' and the 'deformed'). The development of surveillance medicine, which has been present since the early 20th century, however, has compellingly influenced the ways in which we perceive and monitor the health, shape and image of our bodies.

In contemporary times, especially in countries with 'socialised medicine', medical surveillance of the body begins at birth. Every developmental stage of the child's growth and physical functions is closely monitored, controlled, checked, reported, maintained and aligned, plotted and measured against systematically organised medical charts in order to construct and distinguish between the common, the uncommon, the normal and abnormal bodies. This can be seen in the modern day and continued use (since the early 20th Century) of antenatal care, birth notifications, infant welfare clinics and day nurseries. Each of these functions ensures that the early years of child development are closely monitored. The labeling of children as 'normal' or 'abnormal' was not only restricted to their physical and biological functioning, as a child's "psychological growth was construed as inherently problematic, precariously normal. The initial solution was for psychological well-being to be monitored and its abnormal forms identified" (Armstrong).

Under this framework, any child's behaviour that deviates from the mainstream and that does not reflect the average boy or girl next door is automatically placed under the spotlight. The nervous child, the over-sensitive child, the hyperactive child, the neuropathic child, the maladjusted child, the difficult child, the solitary child and the modern day example of the 'special needs' child all emerge as ways of seeing potentially abnormal behaviour leading to a hazardous and problematic childhood.

At every stage of life and development - from childhood, through adolescence to adulthood - young men are encouraged through various forms of surveillance to be responsible for managing their own bodily health and well-being in an attempt to achieve the 'ideal' body. Therefore, I believe that constant surveillance of one's body has a hugely significant effect on young men's body image, identity and behaviour within the world they live. One's body is permanently attached to the judging and monitoring eyes of the public and our identities are inextricably linked to the risk factors and to the avoidance of an abnormal, unhealthy, sick, ill-looking body. British psychology Professor Jane Ogden states:

> *"Surveillance Medicine maps a different form of identity as its monitoring gaze sweeps across innovative spaces of illness potential....Its experiences are inscribed in the progressive realignments implied by emphases on symptoms in the eighteenth century, signs in the nineteenth and early twentieth, and risk factors in the late twentieth century....Its subject and object is the 'risky self."*

To avoid the persistent, judging, eyes of others and too keep our health insurance costs down we construct our bodies (or try to) in order to represent an image of good health, free from illness. Individuals participate in physical activity, they read and analyse the food labels at the grocers (trying to establish what is good and bad), they monitor their alcohol intake (except on a Friday and Saturday night), try to drink lots of water, make regular visits to the doctor at signs of ill health, visit the dentists for annual inspections of decay and force themselves to stop smoking in order to ensure that they limit the risk factors associated with ill health and a sick body. And if that does not work, individuals often use cosmetics, enhancements, replacements, implants, injections, and surgery in order to reconstruct their body and to eliminate the body image of the 'risky self'.

During adolescence, teenage boys' self-awareness and the consciousness of their bodies is significantly heightened in comparison to other stages of development - childhood or adulthood. Self-surveillance of one's body, reinforced by mutual surveillance and 'horizontal surveillance' of peers and friends within the school was used to maintain, monitor and analyse young men's bodily appearance in order to reflect the dominant 'aesthetic-athletic' male represented in popular culture. The effect that mass media has on policing young men's body image is reflected in sociology scholar Peter Corrigan's statement:

*"We are always being scrutinized, we are always being evaluated, our very being is absorbed into the ways in which others look at us: at every moment and in every way we may fail the test of the scrutinizing world."*

Adolescent boys felt suppressed, feeling that they had to live up to masculine ideals and expectations. Young men felt that they could not discuss concerns regarding their bodies, and expressing emotions was associated with weakness, homosexuality and not being a man.

*"The majority of the boys I spoke to feared rejection from friends if they talked about their bodies in the same way girls did. The gender dynamic among the boys gave rise to a complex situation where they feared rejection from peers on the basis of being labeled 'gay' or 'girlie' if they talked about how they or other boys looked."*

The only instance where young men felt that they could freely express themselves and their emotions was while they participated in sports. The sports field or court was an acceptable place for young men to express their emotions, as long as these emotions related to demonstrations of masculinity by exhibiting characteristics of strength, power, heroism and 'machoness'. The ability for young men to express themselves within the sports arena can also be seen within the world of professional sports, whereby sportsman freely celebrate a goal, point, home run or catch with acts of acrobatics, physical gestures, intimacy, emotional release and general exuberant behaviour.

Young men's reluctance to express themselves outside of the sports arena due to the constant surveillance and societal pressure to 'be a man' by hiding their emotions and by hiding any signs of weakness - particularly within the western world - arguably has a negative effect on their health. Emerging research stresses a general reluctance among men - particularly heterosexual men - to express any emotional concerns relating to their body. Given this scenario, it may be that their level of bodily concerns, body dysmorphia and dissatisfaction, have been underestimated. Sociology and psychology studies found that young men negotiated the people who did and did not attain body validation through physical force, strength and pace rather than through talking. Youth researchers have found that boys are schooled in macho-masculinity through participation in playground games which involve physical challenges – such as punch and run, wrestling, fighting and tackling games that demonstrate physical strength and skill.

Young men's bodies, identities, and behaviour are constantly surveilled in order to ensure that they reflect and portray masculine, healthy, and 'aesthetic-athletic' forms. This bodily 'ideal' is reinforced and monitored by the watchful eyes of the media, schools, government, medical establishment, friends and family who subconsciously and consciously influence the way that young men reflect upon their own bodies to ensure that they not only meet societal norms, but that they create physiques that are appealing, desirable and highly accepted.

# NOTES

## CHAPTER ONE    IN PURSUIT OF THE PERFECT BODY

Page : 1    *In an interview with an American bodybuilding website*: Aesthetically Pleasing: Zyzz Shreddedshian Talks With Simplyshredded.com [Updated 2011] Retrieved 9/08/2012.

Page : 2    *'The Sydney Morning Herald'*: _____ (2011, August) The Steroid Generation. The Sydney Morning Herald, p.1.

Page : 2    *American Psychiatrist Harrison Pope, specializing in body image, coined the term 'The Adonis Complex'*: Pope, H.G., Phillips, K.A., & Olivardia, R. (2000). *The Adonis complex: The secret crisis of male body obsession*. Sydney: The Free Press.

Page : 2    *Research shows*: Garner, D., & Kearney-Cooke, A. (1997 January / February). The 1997 body image survey results. *Psychology Today, 30 -36.*

Page : 2    *'The National Survey for Young Australians' reports*: Mission Australia (2007). *National survey of young Australians 2007: key and emerging issues.* Mission Australia.

Page : 3    *'Men's Health' circulation has sky rocketed*: Pope, H.G., Phillips, K.A., & Olivardia, R. (2000). *The Adonis complex: The secret crisis of male body obsession*. Sydney: The Free Press.

Page : 3    *Similar trends have been found on American television*: Parents Television Council (2012, August) *PTC Finds Shocking Spike In Full Nudity on Broadcast TV. Over Five Times More Full Nudity This Season Compared to Last*. Retrieved 10/01/2013 http://www.parentstv.org/ PTC/news/release/2012/0820.asp

Page : 3    *This was evident in a Time Magazine cover*: The Wimpy Recovery: Yes, the economy's getting stronger. So why does it still feel weak? *Time Magazine*, April 2, 2012. (Cover page).

Page : 4    *Research into the bodies of popular boy's toys*: Pope, H.G., Olivardia, R., Gruber & Borowiecki, J. (1999). Evolving Ideals of Male Body Image as Seen Through Action Toys. *International Journal of Eating Disorders*. 26 (1) 65-72. John Wiley & Sons, Inc.

Page : 4    *American Natural body builder: Sadik "Physique" Hadzovic*. (31 January 2012). Retrieved 2012 January http://www.cutandjacked.com/CutAndJacked-Interview-Sadik-Physique-Hadzovic.

Page : 5    *A YMCA study: Central YMCA (2011). A Quarter Of 11 to 16 Year Olds Would Have Cosmetic Surgery To Improve Body Image*, YMCA, United Kingdom.

Page : 9    *Common drugs taken to improve physical appearance include*: Cauchi, A. (2011). Dying for the perfect beach body: Experts warn of the rise of 'bigorexia', *Wentworth Courier*, August 17 pp. 1 & 5.

Page : 9    *In the year 2011 Australian Customs*: Australian Customs (2011). *Customs Reveals Steroid Abuse Is Skyrocketing*. Press Release.


**CHAPTER TWO**        **CRITICAL MOMENTS**

Page : 13    *Erik Erikson (1902-1994)*: Erikson, E.H. (1950). *Childhood and Society*. New York: Norton.

Page : 13    *Erik Erikson (1902-1994)*: Erikson, E.H. (1968). *Identity: Youth and Crisis*. New York: Norton.

Page : 13    *Jean Piaget (1896-1980)*: Piaget, J. (1958). *The Growth of Logical Thinking from Childhood to Adolescence*. Basic Books, New York, NY.

Page : 13    *Urie Bronfenbrenner (1917- 2005)*: Bronfenbrenner, U. (1994). Ecological models of human development. In *International Encyclopedia of Education* (2nd Ed.), Vol. 3. Oxford: Elsevier.

Page : 13    *American sexuality researchers*: Komisaruk, B., Beyer-Flores, C. & Whipple, B. (2006). *The Science of Orgasm*. The Johns Hopkins University Press.

Page : 16    *Documented throughout Western cultures*: Weinke, C. (1998). Negotiating the male body: Men, masculinity, and cultural ideals. *The Journal of Men's Studies*, (6): 255-282.

Page : 16    *American Historian P. Stearns states*: Stearns, P. (2002). Fat History: Bodies and beauty in the Modern West. *Chapter 1: The Turning Point*. pp.9-11. New York University Press.

Page : 18    *Pierre Bourdieu, an influential French sociologist, describes this process*: Bourdieu, P. (1990). *The Logic of Practice* (translated by Richard Nice), Stanford, California: Stanford University Press.

Page : 23    *Sociology scholars*: Patterson, M. & Elliott, R. (2002). Negotiating Masculinities: Advertising and the Inversion of the Male Gaze, Consumption Markets & Culture, (5)3: 231-249.

Page : 24    *American social commentator*: Kimbrell, A. (1993). *The Human Body Shop: The Engineering and Marketing of Life*. Harper Collins, San Francisco.

Page : 26    *American sociologist Jason Whitesel*: Whitesel, J. (2007). Fatvertising: Refiguring Fat Gay Men in Cyberspace. *Limina*, 13, 92-102.

Page : 26    *symbolic of the HIV/AIDS era*: Drummond, M.J. (2005) Men's bodies: listening to the voices of young gay men. *Men and Masculinities*, 7 (3), 270-290.

Page : 27    *Ectomorphic male bodies have often been associated with*: Adams, G., Turner, H. and Bucks, R. (2005). The experience of body dissatisfaction in men, *Body Image*, (2) 271–283. Elsvier.

Page : 27    *Ectomorphic male bodies have often been associated with*: Grogan, S. (2008). *Body Image: Understanding Body Dissatisfaction in Men, Women, and Children*. Routledge.

Page : 27    *These stereotypes can be found among a variety of male populations*: Cone, A., Cass, K. & Ford, J. (2007). Examining body dissatisfaction in young men within a biopsychosocial framework. *Body Image* 5, 183-194. Elsevier.

Page : 28    *what psychologists call a leap in understanding*: McDonald, M.G. (2008). The Nature of Epiphanic Experience. *Journal of Humanistic Psychology* 48: 89. Sage.

Page : 29    *The reflexive body techniques that he used*: Crossley, N. (2005). Mapping Reflexive Body Techniques: On Body Modification and Maintenance. *Body & Society*, 11(1): 1–35. Sage.

Page : 30    *These various popular culture figures and icons*: Pope, H.G., Phillips, K.A., & Olivardia, R. (2000). *The Adonis complex: The secret crisis of male body obsession*. Sydney: The Free Press.

Page : 32    *Incidences of young men being harassed*: Birbeck, D. & Drummond, M. (2005). 'Interviewing, and listening to the voices of, very young children on body image and perceptions of self', *Early Child Development and Care*,175 (6): 579 -596.

Page : 32    *Being too fat, too skinny*: Burrows, L. (2010). Kiwi kids are weetbix kids: Body matters in childhood. *Sport, Education and Society*.

Page : 32    *These young men often grow up*: Rysst, M. & Klepp, I.G. (2012). Looking good and judging gazes: The relationship between body ideals, body satisfaction and body practices among Norwegian men and women. *Health*, 4 (5): 259-267. SciRes.

**CHAPTER THREE**        SEX IN THE CITY

Page : 34    *to accumulate physical capital*: Hakim, C. (2010). "Erotic Capital". *European Sociological Review* 26(5): 499.

Page : 36    *American academic Paul Campos states*: Campos, P.F. (2004). *The Obesity Myth: Why America's Obsession with Weight Is Hazardous to Your Health*. Gotham Books.

Page : 42    *Ty Hamilton, former teammate of*: Hamilton, L. & Coyle, D. (2013). The Secret Race: Inside the Hidden World of the Tour de France. Bantam Books.

Page : 46    *Sports Historian Professor Douglas Booth states*: Booth, D. (2012). *PHSE471 Research Seminar. Context IV: The body*. Otago University.

Page : 50    *What about 'runners' high'*: Boecker, H. (2008). The Runner's High: Opioidergic Mechanisms in the Human Brain. *Cerebral Cortex*, 18: 2523-2531. Advance Access Publication.

Page : 51    *Many exercise scientists would argue that feelings of physiological pleasure*: Dietrich, A. & McDaniel, W.F. (2004). Edoncannabinoids and Exercsie. *Br J Sports Med*; 38:536–541.

Page : 51    *Many exercise scientists would argue that feelings of physiological pleasure*: Booth, D. (2009). Politics and Pleasure: The Philosophy of Physical Education Revisited. *Quest*, 61, 133-153. American Academy of Kinesiology and Physical Education.

Page : 51    *you are what you think*: Hodge, K. (2004). *Sport Motivation: Training Your Mind For Peak Performance*. Reed.

Page : 55    *adolescence is a period of time in ones life where a person searchers for their inner-self*: Burrows, L. & Wright, J. (2004). The discursive production of childhood, identity and health, In Evan, J., Davies, B. & Jan Wright *The Sociology of Physical Education and Health*, 83-95. Routledge.

Page : 55    *adolescence is a period of time in ones life where a person searchers for their inner-self* Erikson, E.H. (1968). *Identity: Youth and Crisis*. New York: Norton.

Page : 57    *In reference to American culture Cain states*: Cain, S. (2012). *Quiet. The Power of Introverts in a World That Can't Stop Talking*. Crown Publishing.

Page : 58    *British sociology scholar Lee Mohanaghan states*: Monaghan, L.F. (2005). Big Handsome Men, Bears and Others: Virtual Constructions of 'Fat Male Embodiment', *Body & Society*, 11: 81, Sage.

Page : 61    These perceived discourses of feminine and gay behavior: Atkinson, M. (2008). Exploring Male Femininity in the 'Crisis': Men and Cosmetic Surgery, *Body & Society*, 14(1): 67–87. Sage.

**CHAPTER FOUR      BEAUTY AND THE BEAST**

Page : 65    *American psychotherapist and social researcher*: Courtenay, W.H. (2000). Constructions of masculinity and their influence on men's well-being: a theory of gender and health. *Social Science and Medicine*, 50 (10), 1385–1401.

Page : 67    *English historian*: Walter, T. (1997). Emotional Reserve and the English Way of Grief. In: *K. Charmaz, G. Howarth and A. Kellehear, eds. The unknown country: death in Australia, Britain and the USA*. Basingstoke, UK: Macmillan, 127–140.

Page : 67    *Sociologists McVittie & Willock*: McVittie, C. & Willock, J. (2006). 'You can't fight windmills': how older men do health, ill health, and masculinities. *Qualitative Health Research*, 16, 788–801.

Page : 67    *"That is to say that to be well…"*: Rosenberg, J.P. (2009). Circles in the surf: Australian masculinity, mortality and grief. *Critical Public Health*, 19:3-4, 417-426.

Page : 68    *"Notions of masculinity like notions of femininity are not static.."*: Courtenay, W.H. (2000). Constructions of masculinity and their influence on men's well-being: a theory of gender and health. *Social Science and Medicine*, 50 (10), 1385–1401.

Page : 68    *French historian and scholar*: Martin, M. (2009). French Masculinities: history, culture and politics. *Medical History*. 53:1.

Page : 69    *Australian historian Marilyn Lake*: Lake, M. (1992). Mission Impossible: How Men Gave Birth to the Australian nation – Nationalism, *Gender and Other Seminal Acts. Gender & History*, 4 (3): 305-322.

Page : 72    *An Australian blogger*: Dann, L. (2010). FUCK AUSTRALIA DAY or "If You Have A Southern Cross Tattoo, Then You're A Racist Cunt", Retrieved 21/02/2014. Betty

Paginated: http://bettypaginated.tumblr.com/post/ 372123358/ fuck-australia-day-or-if-you-have-a-southern

Page : 72   *A English journalist states*: Shad, S. (2012). Australia's Unhealthy Fear of Boat People, Tuesday 8 May, Retrieved 10/12/2012. http://www.guardian.co.uk/commentisfree/2012/may/08/australia-fear-boat-people-asylum-seekers.

Page : 75   *American Psychiatrist Robert Burton*: Burton, W.B. (2005). Aggression and Sport. *Clin Sports Med*, 24, 845-852. Elsevier Saunders.

Page : 77   *Australian and British Education scholars*: Light, R. & Kirk, D. (2000). High School Rugby, the Body and the Reproduction of Hegemonic Masculinity. *Sport, Education and Society*; 5(2):163.

Page : 78   *Their primary purpose was 'to create a universal Tom Brown*: Mangan, J.A. (1998). *The Games Ethic and Imperialism*. London, Frank Cass.

Page : 78   *English sociologist Richard Hoggart*: Hoggart, R. (1957). *The Uses of Literacy: Aspects of Working-class Life with Special Reference to Publications and Entertainments*. London: Chatto and Windus.

Page : 82   *Sociologist Raewyn Connell*: Connell, R.W. (1996) Teaching the Boys: New research on Masculinity, and Gender Strategies for Schools. *Teachers College Record*, (98)2, Winter, Teachers College, Columbia University.

**CHAPTER FIVE**        FROM OBSESSION TO ACCEPTANCE

Page : 88   *"are" bodies and "have" bodies*: Crossley, N. (2001). *The Social Body*. London: Sage.

Page : 89   *given the recent reports published by the Australian Sports Anti-Doping Authority*: Australian Sports Anti-Doping Authority (2013). Retrieved 8 February 2013 http://www.asada.gov.au/media/organised_crime_and_drugs_in_sport.html

Page : 90   *The American Center of Disease Control reports*: Centers for Disease Control and Prevention (2014). Youth Risk Behavior Surveillance – United States, 2013. *MMWR Surveillance Summaries Vol. 63. No. 4.*

Page : 92   *Entertainer Michael Lucas states*: Lucas, M. (2011). Celebrity Interview. In Herman, R. (2011) FOUR-OH! Michael Lucas Enters his Fourth Decade. *Gay Calgary and Edmonton Magazine*, 45.

Page : 95   *Research shows that intrinsic motivation*: Hodge, K. (2004). *Sport Motivation: Training Your Mind For Peak Performance*. Reed.

Page : 96   *Research shows that we are the sum*: Rohn, J. (2012). *My Philosophy For Successful Living*. No Dream Too Big Publishing.

Page : 105   *the human body has often been an 'absent presence'*: Shilling, C. (1993). *The Body and Social Theory*. Sage.

**CHAPTER SIX**          Q & A: SHAPING UP IN THE 21ST CENTURY

Page : 107 *researcher Paul Schilder*: Schilder, P.F. (1935). *The image and appearance of the human body*. London: Kegan Paul, Trench, Trubner.

Page : 107 *Isidore Ziferstein*: Ziferstein, I. (1995). Psychoanalysis and Psychiatry: Paul Ferdinand Schilder 1886-1940. In: Alexander, F., Eisenstein, S., & Grotjahn, M (1966) (eds.): *Psychoanalytic Pioneers*, pp. 457-468, London: New York.

Page : 107 *Psychology Professor Sarah Grogan*: Grogan, S. (2006). Body Image and Health: Contemporary Perspectives. *Journal of Health Psychology*, 11(4) 523–530. Sage

Page : 109 *Psychological studies that interviewed young men*: Grogan, S., & Richards, H. (2002). Body image: Focus group with boys and men. *Men and Masculinities*, 4, 219-232.

Page : 109 *'aesthetic-athletic' male body*: McSharry, S. (2009). Schooled bodies? Negotiating adolescent validation through press, peers and parents. Trentham Books.

Page : 110 *many young men regard themselves as larger or smaller*: Pope, H.G., Phillips, K.A., & Olivardia, R. (2000). *The Adonis complex: The secret crisis of male body obsession*. Sydney: The Free Press.

Page : 110 *Australian research into body image*: O'Dea, J.A. (2010). Studies of obesity, body image and related health issues among Australian adolescents: how can programs in schools interact with and compliment each other? *Journal of Student Wellbeing*, 4(2), 3-16.

Page : 110 *growing up in an era of high modernity*: (Giddens, 1990). Giddens, A. (1990). *The Consequences of Modernity*. Stanford University Press, California.

Page : 110 *The increased scrutiny*: Drummond, M.J. (2003). The meaning of boys' bodies in physical education. *Journal of men's studies*, 11(2): 131-145.

Page : 110 *dramatic increase in the number*: Garner, D., & Kearney-Cooke, A. (1997 January / February). The 1997 body image survey results. *Psychology Today*, 30 -36.

Page : 111 *According to many sociologists in the western world*: Booth, D. (2000). Modern sport: Emergence and experiences. In C. Collins (Eds.), *Sport in New Zealand society* (pp. 45-63). Palmerston North, New Zealand: Dunmore Press.

Page : 111 *Raewyn Connell defines masculinity*: Connell, R.W. (2011). *Raewyn Connell: Masculinities*. Retrieved 21/07/2012: http://www.raewynconnell.net/p/masculinities_20.html.

Page : 111 *Richard Light states*: Light, R. (2008) Learning masculinities in a Japanese high school rugby club. Sport, Education and Society, 13 (2) May, p.163.

Page : 111 *Throughout their school years*: Hickey, C. (2008). Physical education, sport and hyper-masculinity in schools, *Sport, Education and Society*, 13(2): 147-161. Routledge.

Page : 111 *Boys are taught masculinity traits*: Connell, R.W. (2008). Masculinity construction and sports in boys' education: a framework for thinking about the issue, *Sport Education and Society*, 13(2): 131-145. Routledge.

Page : 112 *Men and boys conduct themselves in different ways*: Connell, R.W. (1995). Masculinities. St. Leonards, New South Wales: Allen & Unwin.

Page : 112 *Connell suggests that the dominant masculinity*: Connell, R.W. & Messerschmidt, J.W. (2005). Hegemonic Masculinity: Rethinking the Concept, Gender & Society, 19: 829-859. Sage.

Page : 112 *Majella McSharry, an Irish*: McSharry, S. (2009). *Schooled bodies? Negotiating adolescent validation through press, peers and parents*. Trentham Books.

Page : 114 In some instances young men are taking extreme: Olivardia, R., Pope, H.G., Borowiecki III, J.J., & Cohane, G.H. (2004). Biceps and Body Image: The Relationship Between Muscularity and Self-Esteem, Depression, and Eating Disorder Symptoms. *Psychology of Men & Masculinity*. Educational Publishing Foundation.

Page : 115 *"Schools [placed an] emphasis on hygiene*: Evan, J. & Davies, B. (2004). Endnote: the embodiment of consciousness: Bernstein, health and Schooling. In Evan, J., Davies, B. & Wright, J (Eds.) *Body Knowledge and Control: Studies In The Sociology of Physical Education and Health*, p. 207-217. Routledge: London & New York.

Page : 116 *Sport Sociologist James Cameron states*: Cameron, J. (1993). The sociology of sport. In Perkins, H. & Cushman, G. (Eds.). *Leisure, recreation and tourism*. Auckland: Longman Paul.

Page : 116 *An increased emphasis*: Kirk, D. (1992). Defining Physical Education: *The Social Construction of a School Subject in Post War Britain*, London: Falmer Press.

Page : 117 *Education Professors Evans & Davies state*: Evan, J. & Davies, B. (2004). Endnote: the embodiment of consciousness: Bernstein, health and Schooling. In Evan, J., Davies, B. & Wright, J (Eds.) *Body Knowledge and Control: Studies In The Sociology of Physical Education and Health*, p. 207-217. Routledge: London & New York.

Page : 118 *Sports Historian Douglas Booth argues*: Booth, D. (2000). Modern sport: Emergence and experiences. In C. Collins (Eds.), *Sport in New Zealand society* (pp. 45-63). Palmerston North, New Zealand: Dunmore Press.

Page : 118 *A major concern*: O'Dea, J.A. (2010). Studies of obesity, body image and related health issues among Australian adolescents: how can programs in schools interact with and compliment each other? *Journal of Student Wellbeing*, 4(2), 3-16.

Page : 119 Numerous sociology and psychology research studies: Adams, G., Turner, H. and Bucks, R. (2005). The experience of body dissatisfaction in men, *Body Image*, (2) 271–283. Elsvier.

Page : 119 *These studies found*: Filiault, S.M. & Drummond, J.N. (2010). 'Muscular But Not Roided Out'": Gay Male Athletes And Performance-Enhancing Substances. *International Journal of Men's Health*, 9 (1): 62-81. The Men's Studies Press, LLC.

Page : 119 *English gay magazine 'Attitude'*: Attitude: 5IVE Star, *Attitude Magazine*, May, 2000, p.23. Northern and Shell Network Ltd.

Page : 120 *Participants in Drummond's study*: Drummond, M.J. (2005) Men's bodies: listening to the voices of young gay men. *Men and Masculinities*, 7 (3), 270-290.

Page : 122 *Sociologists Tate and George describe*: Tate, H., & George. R. (2001). The effect of weight loss on body image in HIV-positive gay men. *AIDS Care* 13(2): 163-69.

Page : 122 *'Healthism' as a set of beliefs*: Rose, G. (1992). 'Strategies of prevention: the individual and the population', in M Marmot and P Elliott (Eds.), *Coronary heart disease epidemiology*, p. 311-324.Oxford: Oxford University Press.

Page : 123 *'Healthism' has influenced*: Rose, N. (1990). *Governing the Soul: The Shaping of the Private Self*. London: Routledge.

Page : 123 *Over the last 20 years*: Rysst, M. (2010). "Healthism" and looking good: Body ideals and body practices in Norway. *Scandinavian Journal of Public Health*. 38(5): 71-80. Sage.

Page : 124 *In response to the research question*: Burrows, L. (2010). Kiwi kids are weetbix kids: Body matters in childhood. *Sport, Education and Society*.

Page : 124 *These findings cohere*: Atencio, M. (2006). *'Crunk,' 'cracking and 'choreographies': The place and meaning of health and physical activity in the lives of young people from culturally diverse urban neighbourhoods*. Unpublished PhD thesis, University of Wollongong, Australia. Beausoleil, N. (2008). *Meanings of health, physical activity and schooling in Newfoundland and New Brunswick youths' narratives*. Paper presented a: the Australian Association for Research in Education Conference, University of Queensland, Brisbane, Australia. Shea, J. (2006). *"An apple a day keeps the doctor away": Immigrant youth in St. John's, New Foundland and Labrador and their constructions of health and fitness*. Unpublished PhD thesis. Memorial University of Newfoundland, St John's Newfoundland, Canada.

Page : 125 *Contemporary sociologist David Lyon*: Lyon, D. (2007). *Surveillance Studies: An Overview*. Polity.

Page : 125 *Governments and law*: Armstrong, D. (1995). The rise of surveillance medicine. *Sociology of Health & Illness*, 17 (3): 393- 404.

Page : 125 *Together with several contemporary scholars*: Gallagher, C. (2003). CCTV and Human Rights: the Fish and the Bicycle? An Examination of Peck V. United Kingdom, *In Surveillance and Society: CCTV Special* (Eds.) Norris, McCahill and Wood 2(2/3): 270-292.

Page : 126 *Firstly, society's awareness*: Stanely, J. and Steinhardt, B. (2003). "Bigger Monster, Weaker Chains: The Growth of an American Surveillance Society". *American Civil Liberties Union*. New York, January.

Page : 126 *the rise of the obesity epidemic*: Burrows, L. (2011). Thinking with attitude, In S. Brown (Ed.) *Issues and Controversies in Physical Education: Policy, Power and Pedagogy*. Pearson. Burrows, L. & Wright, J. (2004). The discursive production of childhood, identity and health, In Evan, J., Davies, B. & Jan Wright *The Sociology of Physical Education and Health*, 83-95. Routledge.

Page : 126 *And, thirdly, the increased power*: Shapiro, M.J. (2005). Every Move You Make: Bodies, Surveillance, and Media, *Social Text Summer*, 23(83): 21-34.

Page : 126 *In an interview with The Guardian*: The Guardian (2014) NSA Whistleblower Edward Snowden Interview. Retrieved 12/04/2015 http://www.theguardian.com/world/video/2013/jun/09/nsa-whistleblower-edward-snowden-interview-video

Page : 128 *In the last 5-years scholars*: Weitzer, R. & Tuch, S.A. (2006). Perceptions of Racial Profiling: Race, Class, and Personal Experience. Criminology Volume 40, Issue 2, 435 – 456, May 2002.

Page : 129 *Sociologist John Hargreaves*: Hargreaves, J. (1986). *Sport, Power and Culture: A Social and Historical Analysis of Popular Sports in Britain*. Polity Press: Cambridge.

Page : 129 *Prominent Sociologist Michel Foucault*: Foucault, M. (1982). 'Technologies of the Self', In Luther H. Martin, Huck Gutman and Patrick H. Hutton (Eds.) *Technologies of the Self: A Seminar with Michel Foucault*, p. 16–49. Amherst: The University of Massachusetts Press, 1988.

Page : 130 *"inculcating desires*: Rose, N. (1999). *Powers of Freedom: reframing political thought*. Cambridge: Cambridge University Press.

Page : 131 *The development of surveillance medicine*: Armstrong, D. (1995). The rise of surveillance medicine. *Sociology of Health & Illness*, 17 (3): 393- 404.

Page : 132 *British Psychology Professor*: Ogden, J. (1995). Psychosocial theory and the creation of the risky self, *Social Science and Medicine*, 40 (3): 409-15.

Page : 133 *The effect that mass media*: Corrigan, P. (1997). The Sociology of Consumption: an introduction. London: Sage.

Page : 133 *"The majority of the boys*: McSharry, S. (2009). *Schooled bodies? Negotiating adolescent validation through press, peers and parents*. Trentham Books.

Page : 133 *The sports field*: Connell, R.W. (2008). Masculinity construction and sports in boys' education: a framework for thinking about the issue, *Sport Education and Society*, 13(2): 131-145. Routledge.

Page : 134 *Emerging research stresses*: Cleary, A. (2005). 'Death Rather than Disclosure: struggling to be a real man' in Irish *Journal of Sociology*, 14(2): 155-176.

Page : 134 *As other youth researchers*: Kehily, M.J. & Nayak, A. (1997). Lads and Laughter: humour and the production of heterosexual hierarchies, *Gender and Education*, 9(1): 69-87.